On Borrowed Time

Living With Hemodialysis

By Samuel B. Chyatte, M.D.

Medical Economics Company **MEBD** Book Division
Oradell, New Jersey 07649

Design by JoAnne Cassella

ISBN 0-87489-213-9

Medical Economics Company
Oradell, New Jersey 07649

Printed in the United States of America

To Helen
and to Michelle, Gerri, Scott, and Brett

Contents

Foreword

In Chapter 21, "We All Must Die," Sam Chyatte wrote that he wanted a swift and relatively easy death. His death—on July 31, 1978—came exactly as he had wished.

In life, he was husband, father, physician, patient. Though he tried hard to keep these roles distinct, he couldn't. Each, in some way, influenced the others. This, too, is obvious in the book. As you read it, you'll see that his being a patient greatly influenced Sam's family and professional life. Having strong family ties helped him to empathize with his patients and to understand how their disabilities affected their family relationships.

Sam's disease changed his professional life in another way. In 1975, when he came down with end-stage renal disease as a complication of a long-standing chronic disorder, he directed his work toward helping ESRD patients. He did this for two reasons: First, it was a matter of professional interest. At the time, no one was working with rehabilitation of ESRD patients, and Sam felt that this was a new, vital area that needed to be studied and researched. Second, specializing in ESRD rehabilitation was a way to help him cope with his own disease process. On Borrowed Time is an outgrowth of that activity.

As you'll quickly see, the book is extremely personal. At times, you may get the uncomfortable feeling that you're intruding upon Sam's personal life and his most private thoughts. This is how Sam wanted his book to affect its readers. He wanted the layperson, professional, and paraprofessional worker in ESRD not only to gain *intellectual* insight into the disease as it affects a patient. He wanted them to *feel* the problem as well.

The ESRD patient who reads On Borrowed Time will identify with Sam and many of the circumstances he portrays, and thereby, Sam hoped, will understand, accept, and cope with the ESRD process. This is the beginning of rehabilitation—Sam's specialty. Through this book, so long as ESRD patients are helped by it, Sam's work will continue far longer in years than any ordinary man's.

He couldn't have a more fitting memorial.

Barry J. Rosenbaum, M.D.
Atlanta Nephrology Referral Center
Decatur, Georgia

Publisher's Notes

As both physician and patient, Dr. Chyatte knew from both viewpoints what it is like to have and to cope with end-stage renal disease.

After 12 years with diabetes mellitus, Dr. Chyatte developed chronic kidney disease. (About one-fourth of all renal patients are diabetics.) As his kidney disease inevitably progressed to what is called the end stage (the last stage of deterioration before complete kidney failure), Dr. Chyatte was faced with a choice: Death then, or dialysis. He delayed death with dialysis for two and a half years. Dr. Chyatte died on July 31, 1978, just a few weeks before he was to see first proofs of this book.

Dr. Chyatte was not just a physician who happened to be on dialysis. He continued his medical practice during his last years, working perhaps harder than ever, but with a new focus. He concentrated on rehabilitating renal patients, helping them cope with their disease. This book is just one part of that work. He was professor of rehabilitation medicine at Emory University School of Medicine, clinical director of Emory's Center for Rehabilitation Medicine, project director of the center's Renal Rehabilitation Project, and director of the university's Regional Rehabilitation Research and Training Center.

Dr. Chyatte obviously had the credentials and personal experience to write about ESRD. As you read his book, you'll quickly become aware that he also possessed—to a remarkable degree—the sensitivity to write about the human dimensions of ESRD: The thoughts and feelings, the trials and triumphs of patients and their families.

Almost every chapter of On Borrowed Time expresses a zest for life. Throughout the book, you'll find Dr. Chyatte saying that things are getting better, hoping that someday renal patients will be free of at least some of the limitations that ESRD and dialysis presently impose on them. His optimism, however, was tempered with realism. With his manuscript, he sent us this poem:

> Time no longer is my friend.
> I cannot wait for its decisions.
> Its passage does not heal my wounds.
> Time is unyielding.
>
> The future has a past tense,
> For it holds only what is already known.
> I know what I do not wish to know.
> The future is a painful memory.
>
> Evening steals my light.
> Will morning bring me more?
> Tomorrow's tomorrow is a question.
> What shall I do until there is none?

Introduction

More than 40,000 people survive today because artificial kidneys keep them alive. These people have end-stage renal disease (ESRD); their own kidneys don't work anymore. Artificial kidneys are machines that clean—or dialyze—the blood of ESRD patients.

Places where this cleaning is done—dialysis centers—must meet medical and governmental standards. There are no standards for dealing with people, however. Perhaps physicians, nurses, and technicians ought to experience the diseases their patients have. But since, luckily for them, most health professionals don't undergo such difficult learning experiences, they can only guess at what their patients may be feeling or thinking. This book should help medical personnel gain that insight.

As a physician and an ESRD patient, I know both worlds. It has been an enlightening yet humbling experience. It has enabled me to write not just about the disease, but about people who have it. It has helped me to see ESRD's medical complications through the eyes of the patient, not the doctor. Along the way, I have suggested some helpful adapting and coping guides for patients' families. ESRD isn't a disease of the patient alone; it's a problem that affects the entire family.

In 1960, when the artificial kidney was first used on a routine basis for maintenance therapy, patients spent from 12 to 16 hours on the machine for each treatment. They were kept alive, but could not do much else. Since then, technology advanced, and dialysis machines became more efficient and less cumbersome. Now, with treatment shortened to between three and five hours, patients have time to do other things with their lives. In addition, people can rent or purchase units and dialyze in the comfort of their own homes on their own schedules. Portable units that allow greater mobility are available and are being improved.

With these advances, ESRD patients have become people again. They have a reasonable life expectancy. Some have been surviving for more than 10 years on artificial kidney support. Their problems now revolve around competing in and getting along with a normal world. They still have medical problems, of course, but these now share the spotlight with human concerns.

Medical technology is full of promises for ESRD patients: adsorbents, taken by mouth, to reduce the need for dialysis; smaller, portable machines, some that can be worn; increasing success with kidney transplants. Each tomorrow will be better. You've got to get there to enjoy it.

Samuel B. Chyatte, M.D.

1

Kidney Disease and Its Treatment

ESRD is a condition in which the kidneys no longer perform their life-sustaining function of controlling the body's fluid and electrolyte balance. Waste materials accumulate, and death is certain to follow unless proper treatment is instituted. This is what ESRD means medically.

But to patients with chronic renal failure, ESRD means deciding not to buy a new pair of shoes, because what's left of life is too short to get enough use out of them. It's wondering how your spouse will cope when you're gone. It's experiencing intense, unrelenting itching and feeling your skin stretched and taut with edema. It's being unable to bend over to tie your shoes without getting short of breath. To me, it was deadening fatigue. To all of us, it's hopelessness, depression, confusion, and helplessness. It's life in disarray. It's welcoming death as a solution. Then, when you feel you can no longer go on, you're offered a chance to live again— renal transplantation or dialysis therapy.

On Borrowed Time: Living With Hemodialysis

Many diseases can impair kidney function and lead to chronic renal failure. High blood pressure and diabetes may cause generalized damage to parts of the body, injuring the kidneys in the process. They're attacked more directly by glomerulonephritis and pyelonephritis. Other disorders, such as polycystic kidney disease, are inherited. It's important to understand your own particular set of problems. Discuss them with your doctor. Don't suppose that if you don't talk about your disease, it will vanish. Ignorance can lead to even greater troubles.

Let's go into some detail about what happens when a patient learns that he or she has kidney disease. The general statements I'll make I've drawn largely from personal experience, but also from patient interviews and from what I've read in medical and psychological journals.

The impact of kidney disease may strike suddenly, as it did in my case. It was about five years before actual renal failure that I learned I was in trouble. I had been diabetic for about 12 years and always knew that renal disease could develop from diabetes. I remember that first visit to my physician. It was cold in the examining room, but the goose bumps I felt arose as well from fear. It seemed silly, but I passed time reading the framed diplomas and listening to the sounds of people passing by the door.

Helen—my wife—had to insist that I come. Physicians, perhaps more than most other people, don't like to be patients, but there I sat, stripped to the waist and stripped of whatever power a physician is presumed to have over disease. I was a patient. I was defenseless, frightened, and more than a little apprehensive.

I had decided to come to Paul because I didn't know him very well. Detachment, I thought, would make it easier for my doctor—and me—to be matter-of-fact and objective. Paul had recently started private practice. Before that, he and I served on the same hospital staff. We had different specialties and didn't see each other often. He had a reputation for integrity, intelligence, and competence, and, whenever I met him, I found him easygoing and pleasant. I was satisfied with my choice. By the time the door opened, I was also glad to see another human being.

Paul was pleasant, competent, and frank. He examined me physically after taking the history of my 12 years of diabetes mellitus, the early changes in my vision, my hypertension, and the pain in my hands and arms. After chest X-rays, electrocardiograms, a few laboratory tests, and other bodily intrusions, he asked me to return at the end of the next week, when he would have the lab results, so that we could discuss my situation.

It was a long week. I already knew I was in trouble, but I didn't know just how deeply and I worried a lot about it. I already knew the limits to what could be done, but, like everyone else, I wanted someone to tell me that I'd be cured. I was early for the Friday appointment.

Paul pointed out that diabetes is a long-term illness that gradually breaks down a whole host of systems in the body and that I would need long-term care, with special attention to diet, infections, regulation of life-style, and work load. He noted that my nervous system, eyes, and kidneys were already impaired. These facts weren't alarming—I had already guessed that this was the case.

I nervously joked—perhaps first to test my voice—about deteriorating and becoming a charity patient at the hospital. Then I looked directly at Paul and asked, "How long? How much longer will I be able to practice? Ten years?" I put it in terms of work; I wasn't able to think yet about my life being so limited. I had calculated it several times during the previous week and felt that 10 years was a reasonable estimate. I felt I was logical, calm, and confident. His brief answer was shattering. "No," he said. "I think it's more like five."

These easy words confounded all my logic, calm, and confidence. Thoughts raced in a dozen desperate directions. I rushed into my home, brushed past Helen, and disappeared into my bedroom. Helen wasn't far behind; she had read the terror in my face. I wanted to be calm and reassuring, but instead I held her and cried, "I'm going to die. He gave me five years to live."

I spent most of that weekend in bed, drenching my pillow with tears. I was in deep depression; looking back, there is no other way to describe it, though I wouldn't have called it that at the time. I can't remember even wondering how Helen felt. I didn't consider telling the children. It was to be years before they'd learn how close I was to death. By Monday, I had regained some control and returned to work. I had suppressed the emotional reaction; it surfaced only occasionally from then on.

When you first learn that you have kidney disease, you probably go through two distinct reactions. The first is more intellectual; you ask yourself questions like: "What does that mean? Can it be cured? Will I be able to work? Will I die? If I die, what'll happen to my family? Who'll care for the children?" These questions try to uncover facts about the unknown. They pass through your mind, with some urgency, even before you can ask them aloud. Many have no answers, at least not just yet.

The second reaction is one you feel, an emotional confusion and depression that comes when you realize that the body you took for granted is not to be taken for granted anymore. There's a sense of impending doom. You feel lost and very much alone. You want to do something, but you just don't know what.

While you are in this state, your mind doesn't work properly. You don't receive information well and you don't process it well. You don't hear half of what the doctor tells you. Some key words will register, but a good many details won't. Your doctor, for example, may say that you have a 10 per cent chance of dying in the next year. You hear only that you may die, and you don't remember anything he told you about your disease.

4

The person who suddenly goes into kidney failure has little opportunity to adapt. For most of us, the process is slower. When the initial shock wears off, we realize that we're not in immediate danger. After all, it took time to get to the end-stage. We adapt and keep functioning.

Adaptation is an important mechanism that protects us as our health fails. Little by little, we learn to cope with our illness. The problem is that we sometimes continue to adapt while becoming progressively worse. Often we put off seeing the doctor because we are still "getting along O.K." And, when we finally see him, we plead for "just a little more time" before going on an artificial kidney.

When the time for dialysis arrives, you're never quite ready. Many fellow patients have told me that they talked their doctors out of it for a while. Now that they have crossed over to the other side, they see how foolish they were and agree that they should have begun dialysis earlier. It's the emotional impact of that step that kept them from doing so. They felt that to go on dialysis is to surrender to the disease, to become dependent on a machine for life, and to undergo a complex set of emotional and physical adjustments that life on the machine brings with it.

Transplant patients generally have gone the dialysis route first and have experienced these reactions. But transplantation brings its own problems. First, although very few people die of it, it would be naive not to worry about the surgery itself. The transplant patient also lives with the fear, sometimes for years, that the transplanted kidney will be rejected by the body. All of the pros and cons have to be considered (see Chapter 7). The decision is difficult.

ESRD is a whole new way of life, but you adjust and you can thrive. You can tell yourself, "I have a chronic illness that I can control. It's tough; I feel sorry for myself and the people around me, but we're all going to make it." As people with ESRD survive longer and do better, it would be a shame not to be around to see what's coming next.

5

2 Renal Failure and Your Feelings

You get tired. Getting up, getting showered, and getting dressed are enough to tire you out for the rest of the day. Fatigue is common to people with kidney failure, as are the following symptoms and emotions. Poisons build up in your body because your kidneys don't clear them out. As a result, the chemistry of your body and its cells becomes more and more disturbed, and your body just doesn't work right. Your red blood cells are being destroyed faster than usual, and you don't make these cells as fast as you used to. You become anemic, and your cells aren't getting the oxygen they need. In a sense, your blood has "thinned." The face that looks back at you in the mirror is pale, grayish yellow.

Your ankles may be swollen. Perhaps the swelling goes higher—into your legs—and sometimes it develops in your lungs. If your lungs get involved, when you lie down to sleep at night you may get short of breath.

Everyone seems to bother you. You are short-tempered

and irritable. Children get on your nerves. Maybe it's because you don't sleep well at night. You're tired, but you sleep only for short stretches and wake up restless.

Your stomach bothers you. It always feels upset. You have a lot of gas. Your appetite is diminished. Food doesn't appeal to you as it once did.

Your mind doesn't seem to work right. You can't remember things that have always been familiar to you. Sometimes you are too confused to work out problems. Reading is difficult because you can't concentrate.

Sitting in a chair has become a problem. You shift position, but your legs just can't get comfortable. Perhaps the soles of your feet burn and your muscles twitch.

Sex is less interesting. You may have become impotent, but you're so tired you may not even care.

And that itching, like a family of fire ants picnicking on your skin, is driving you crazy.

Some of these symptoms—the headaches, confusion, sluggish thought and speech, apathy, difficulty with memory and concentration—are more troubling than others. It should help you—and your friends and family—to realize that these symptoms are due to the effects the toxic materials in your blood have on your brain. They appear just before or early on in dialysis, which usually corrects them.

A sick person may think that his suffering is unique, that no one has gone through the same problems. This is not true. There is a common thread to illness. It helps to realize that others have experienced the same problems and that others will in the future.

I was better prepared for sickness than most people. For 10 years I had taught medical students the psychology of disability, and treated patients with spinal-cord injuries, strokes, amputations, and other catastrophic disorders. I was well aware that I hadn't been singled out to suffer. As my disease advanced, however, I was shocked to find that I was living through things I had lectured about. I knew, before, that they were true. Now I was experiencing them, and that is quite different.

Even though I understood the predictable stages of illness, I was constantly amazed by each new stage. Knowing what to expect didn't change my behavior one bit. I did all the things a patient is expected to do; I was a textbook case.

If you are so tired that you can't speak in whole sentences, don't think you're the only one who feels this way. As your muscles cramp, you're not alone either. If you ask, "Why me? What am I being punished for?" rest assured there are thousands of people also asking those questions.

Psychologists have described five stages that the chronically ill or disabled go through as they adjust to their conditions. They are: 1) denial, 2) depression, 3) changing images, 4) rationalization, and 5) accommodation. This may sound complicated, but you don't need a Ph.D. to recognize these stages as you read on.

Denial is exactly what it says it is. You deny the implications of your condition because you can't cope just yet. Suppose you cut your finger. First, you're a bit upset, then you put your finger under running water, smear antiseptic on it, and wrap a bandage around it. Only occasionally does a pain remind you that you're hurt. But if you cut off your leg, you can't accept the loss so casually. You can't accept so significant a change in your body and your life all at once. When you deny some of its problems, you shield yourself from the full impact of the catastrophe. The same is true of kidney disease. First comes the shock of learning that your kidneys are failing. Then you see that nothing much about your life has suddenly or drastically changed, and you say, "What am I worried about? I'm still O.K." For a while, at least, you deny it is a real problem.

But the disease progresses. Eventually you are faced with dialysis and dependency—dependency on a machine and on the people who run it. For people who don't like to be waited upon, dialysis may be unbearable. If you're like this,

9

you may deny your illness by ignoring your diet. You may not limit your fluids. You may skip your medications. When you're on edge at home or work, you say, "It's nothing." All these actions can be denial.

Still, denial isn't all bad. If I were to skip the denial stage, I'd say to myself, "I'm at the end-stage. I know what that means: I'm going to die. There's no use in doing *anything.*" Instead, I put my illness out of my mind—deny it—and say, "I'm not so sick. I'm not bedridden. There's a lot I can accomplish." That's useful denial. I'm sick, but I keep going. I just push away the implications of my illness.

In time, reality creeps through your denial; you begin to deal with your problem, and you become depressed. You realize that you will die or have to depend on a machine for life. Fears surface, self-pity comes out, and you grieve for your loss. Yet, depression and tears seem to be a mechanism that restores the grieved to normalcy. Most widows, for example, cry long and hard before they resume more normal lives. The person who doesn't experience depression is stuck in the denial stage and never comes to grips with himself.

Depression can be destructive. Though it's a normal reaction, it may become severe enough to bring you to the edge of suicide. Even at such an extreme, you're dealing with your situation in a way that is consistent with *how you know it.* How can you know you will one day feel so much better?

As you begin to see that you are better, that you'll survive, you begin to climb out of your depression. And as you improve, you begin to change your self-image. While you were more acutely ill, you probably lost the image of yourself that you had built over the years. As you grew from childhood, you learned what you could do—what you were good at and what you weren't—chose what you wanted to do, defined yourself, created your self-image. Illness destroyed that self-image, and now you have to develop a new one. You have to learn all over again what you can do, what your limits are. You learn a new you.

Gradually, you begin to rationalize. You say, "You know, I enjoy life more than I used to. I never took time for it before. Now I can." You start to look at the brighter, positive side of things. You see the dialysis center, for example, not as a place just for treatment, but as a place where you meet people you have come to like.

The final stage is accommodation. After learning who you are and your new capacities and limitations, you are at peace with yourself. You are ready to deal with the world from a firm foundation. You've come full circle: Just as you grew from the unclear self-image of childhood, you have now grown from the unclear self-image of chronic illness.

Once you've come to accept your condition, you're not through with feelings and emotions. You've got to come to terms emotionally with dialysis, too. Some psychologists divide the reactions to dialysis into three stages. When you start dialysis you are at a low point, perhaps near death. Dialysis brings you "back to life." You get better, feel better, and enter a honeymoon period when everything looks great. This period may begin three weeks after you start dialysis and lasts perhaps six months.

After the honeymoon, a period of discouragement and disenchantment follows. Often it comes when you try to resume a normal life. You find things are different, and you are discouraged. You feel sad and helpless.

Finally, there is long-term adaptation to your new life. During this time, you will sometimes be confident and happy, sometimes discouraged and depressed. As you go through these shifts in feelings, you may wonder whether you're normal. All people have some emotional swings— elation and depression, fearlessness and anxiety—whether healthy or not. That doesn't change. ESRD just intensifies our moods. So, whether you're normal or not depends upon what you were like before ESRD.

All of us end-stage patients have been near death, some closer to it than others. Although ESRD is no longer thought of as a terminal illness—it's a chronic disease that can be managed—the future is uncertain. You naturally have some anxiety about survival and about the quality of your life if you survive. Anxiety and depression are sometimes disguised. How do you recognize them?

Anxiety is a feeling of uneasiness or apprehension, a sense of something wrong, though frequently you can't figure out what that something is. It may be accompanied by sweating, a pounding pulse or heartbeat, irritability, or fatigue. Anxiety makes it hard to concentrate, make decisions, or sit still. Ordinary routines, such as shopping or writing a letter, may be impossible. All of us have anxiety at times, but the patient who is constantly anxious needs help.

Depression is a down feeling, otherwise described as sadness, discouragement, or gloom. Nothing is going right, and maybe you don't even care anymore. Your appetite for everything—food, work, pleasure, sex—decreases. Sleep doesn't come easily. Even your speech slows down. Not many ESRD patients become so depressed that they try suicide, but some are suspected of deliberately bringing on death by ignoring their diets and fluid restrictions, or by not taking their medications.

If you have anxieties that trouble you greatly, or feelings that go to unmanageable extremes, it's smart to look for help. Don't let a problem interfere with your medical progress. An unhappy or disturbed person responds less well to dialysis than does a happy person and may be inclined to disregard his doctor's advice.

You can approach your physician or nurse first. If neither picks up your SOS, seek out a dialysis center social worker, who is trained to listen. There are other professionals who can help: family, sex, or rehabilitation counselors; rabbis, ministers, psychologists, or psychiatrists. Needing help doesn't mean you're crazy. Very few ESRD patients are, but almost all of us now and then have problems that require someone else's help. And that's normal.

3

Renal Failure and Your Friends

We ESRD patients have to realize that our disease affects other people. As we go through the illness, family and friends are going through changes also. Their problems are different, of course, but real and important. Patients tend to be introspective. They think a great deal about themselves, their bodies, and their survival. Family and friends have watched and worried too, as your condition worsened. They wondered whether you'd live, how they could manage without you, who'd pay the bills or do the shopping.

There's even a typical pattern to their reactions. For instance, when you first became so ill that you had to be hospitalized, your family and your friends clustered around. People called to ask how they could help. Even your employer was kind and understanding. Everyone was concerned. Aunt Maude, who hadn't been in touch for 10 years, called to ask about you. You were the center of attraction. Your every wish seemed to bring an immediate response.

On Borrowed Time: Living With Hemodialysis

When you came home, though, the attention dwindled. Fewer and fewer people called. The family, which had marshaled all its emotional and financial resources during the initial crisis, returned to the business of everyday life.

Clearly, here—in everyday life—changes have taken place. Once you played certain roles: breadwinner or homemaker, parent-figure, spouse, lover, or keeper of the checkbook. But if you no longer work, you're no longer the breadwinner. Someone else now writes the checks. Someone else takes care of the lawn or has become the meal maker.

You used to be at the center of household decisions: Do we buy a second car? Which bills do we pay first? Can we afford a vacation this year? While you were ill, others carried all the weight of those decisions.

As you return to better health, you should recapture some of these roles. Otherwise, the new patterns become fixed. And, if you're not careful, so does your sick role. In other words, you remain helpless.

In most cases, ESRD patients get well enough to take up responsibilities again. But some people enjoy being helpless. Others take advantage of their illness.

One young man I knew said he could walk for miles, climb stairs, party, make love, and do whatever he wanted to do, even drink. I asked him if he wanted help getting a job. "I don't want a job," he said. "That'd take up too much of my time." He had found an easy life—a regular disability check and only one responsibility: dialysis three times a week.

Another man found that his family, who, it seemed, had ignored him when he was well, now waited on him hand and foot. He didn't want to lose that by getting too well!

The degree to which a patient with ESRD recaptures the roles that others have taken up may be considered the degree to which he is rehabilitated. Some of you will regain your functions, others may not. If you don't, it's no reason to think you're a failure. The onetime laborer who can't read or write will be much less likely to find employment than the man who owns his own business. That's not failure for want of effort; it's circumstance. All each of us can do is avoid the trap of enjoying our illness.

Some relatives and friends may react to your illness in peculiar ways. Their reactions vary according to their own problems or fears. Some may be stoic and keep a stiff upper lip; some become awkward and don't know what to say; others become overly concerned. When I told some of my relatives the unpleasant statistics involved in ESRD, they answered, "Don't talk like that; everything will be O.K." They couldn't handle it.

Friends surprised me. You expect close friends to see you through it all, and casual friends to have only a passing interest. It didn't always work out that way. Some were fantastic. They visited us and took us out, even though that meant hauling me around in a wheelchair. One friend, a physician, forced himself on me at a time when I didn't want to talk to anyone. It was he who got me to turn the corner out of depression and back into an active life.

Some people, close friends, didn't call, visit, or write. Others, casual friends or acquaintances, came by and kept in touch. After a while I discovered what was going on. My close friends who seemed to ignore me couldn't express their feelings. The casual friends who were so concerned about me had gone through some things in their own lives that had sensitized them to others in distress. One had a retarded child about whom I didn't know. Another who was also helpful had lost a child many years before.

Seems that, when you fall ill and stay ill, people feel sorry for you. Sometimes, the sorrier they feel, the more it makes them feel vulnerable. They're afraid something as serious will happen to them. They can't face you, because they're so threatened by what has happened to you.

Also, many people back off from what is strange or different, and, let's face it, you *are* strange to other people; they've never experienced anything like what you've gone through. A leg cast isn't uncommon; people can relate to that. But it's hard for people to understand the chemistry and complications of kidney disease.

With all these problems that people have in dealing with your illness, what happens when they come to visit is that *you* need to cheer *them* up. Keep a humorous perspective on your problems. Instead of complaining about your food, for example, you might say, "Want to stay for dinner? We're having four ounces of salt-free hamburger, half a baked potato, and a green lettuce salad with lemon juice. On the side you get a half-cup of coffee and an orange-free fruit cup." That tells your plight and leaves them smiling.

In general, talk about things your visitors are interested in, and things you used to talk about before you became ill: sports, politics, vacations. People will be more comfortable with you and will be readier to return.

People, by and large, will relate to you according to the image you project. Strangers will not know of your ESRD problems and will view you as they would anyone else. Friends will know of your problems, but they'll like you or dislike you according to what you do, what you say, and how you make them feel. If you project the image of a sick, dependent person, that's how you'll be treated.

Your friends will readily accommodate their visiting and entertaining to meet your needs, but they don't know how. Let them know. If they invite you over at a time that's bad for you because of dialysis, tell them why you can't come. If they make a dish you can't eat, tell them why and offer an alternative. "We're planning a ground meat, noodles, and tomato sauce dish," one friend called to tell us. "Just a hamburger and noodles, please," we had to say.

Of course, you can't go out for pizza and beer—those two "kidney busters." You just have to explain why.

Now that you know all about yourself and everyone else, you're ready to meet the world. Don't let it go by without you.

4 Telling the Children

You know you're going to die. It may be years before it happens, but not very many. How do you tell your children? I didn't tell mine until actual renal failure. I remember my children's apprehension when I entered the hospital for the vascular surgery that I needed to get ready for hemodialysis. The youngest one, Brett, later told me he was afraid I wouldn't come home again. He was frightened when he came to visit. After he played with the electric bed and the remote-control TV, he eased up a bit, but he still wasn't himself. The older children are generally more reserved, but they, too, were subdued.

Since my oldest two were teenagers, I decided they should know the facts. I sat them down and told them that my kidneys were failing and that I was dying. I perhaps should have displayed more optimism. However, I've never been an optimist, so it wouldn't have been in keeping with my personality and wouldn't have had the ring of truth about it. My younger daughter, Gerri, couldn't sleep that night. Michelle became pale and silent. It was one of the most painful experiences I've ever endured.

Shortly after I had told the girls, I told my older son, Scott. He had just gone to bed, when I came into his room. Somehow, I couldn't turn on the light. First, I touched him, but the tears began to fall, so I walked over and looked out his window. Then I told him what was happening and I asked him to be a model for his younger brother. When I left, I heard him cry. He hadn't cried since he was a little boy. I don't know who hurt more, he or I.

I've never been able to tell Brett, who was seven when this began.

Was I right to tell them so much, or was I trying to relieve my guilty feelings caused by my deserting them? Did they feel that I was abandoning them? That I was destroying our family? After all, I had just destroyed their security. I had made their lives frightening. I only know that the children reflected my moods and behavior. My irritability drove them from me. My depression depressed them. My restoration has seemed to restore them.

Someone asked me at a renal conference, "How are the children of dialysis patients affected?" My answer must have seemed a bit vague. I said, "The children will react as their parents do. If the parent complex copes with the problem well, the children will also cope. If the parent complex does not cope, the children will not." I used the term "parent complex," because both the husband and the wife will influence the children, and each spouse must deal with himself and his partner in order for the home situation to remain stable and secure.

There are many ways for a marriage to work under normal circumstances. In some arrangements, the husband has certain roles (breadwinner, taker to baseball games, checkbook keeper), and the wife has others (homemaker, carpool driver, gardener). In other arrangements, both husband and wife are employed, both do housework, both cook, and both handle money. If everyone is satisfied, one particular arrangement doesn't make more sense than another.

Children function best when they know the rules. If they grow up with Dad doing the cooking and Mom going to the office and everybody being happy about it, they'll be satisfied. But when ESRD disrupts family roles, it changes the rules of the game. The children don't know where they fit or what the roles are.

Also, each of us has personality traits, habits and ways of approaching things. Our children learn our ways without thinking about them. They identify us in roles and images. Renal disease changes behavior. I remember one incident for which I can never forgive myself. It was early in dialysis, and I could just barely get myself to a standing position. Ordinarily, Helen wouldn't have left me alone, but she had been at my side for weeks without a break and she had to get out briefly. I lay on my bed upstairs, while two of the teenagers watched TV in the basement playroom. I wanted something, though I can't even remember now what it was. I called for help. No answer. I called and called. No answer. I became enraged. What if I were really in trouble? Where the devil were they? By this time I was furious—furious out of all proportion to the original issue.

Finally, Scott heard my bellowing and raced upstairs. I was so angry, I hit him with my cane on his elbow. I didn't intend to hit him, but I did. I hadn't raised a hand to him since he was old enough to talk to. "Go to hell," he screamed. "I don't care if you die. I'm not coming up here again." I was so irrationally angry I couldn't apologize.

His mother packed his arm in ice when she came home. For days Scott carried his arm as if it were broken, glaring at me whenever we met. He refused to acknowledge any healing. Finally, we took him for X-rays. He became flustered when the secretary asked him what happened. Apparently, he was torn between the embarrassment of telling what really happened, and the alternative of making up a story. After the X-ray showed no damage, he returned to normal. He had been punishing me for hitting him, though I don't think he knew that. When I returned to my more normal personality, one of my daughters told Helen, "It's nice to have Daddy back again." I was driving them all away, but I simply couldn't help myself.

Reactions to ESRD among children vary in part in relation to the ages. A two-year-old and an 18-year-old obviously see things quite differently. In addition to age, there are other influencing factors: interactions among children in the same family, friends and other outside influences, and even events on TV or other media. Dialysis patients on TV are often displayed as near death or with some horrible problem, and children—and patients—often accept this drama as an accurate portrayal of real life.

It is difficult to look at ESRD through your child's eyes, but, if you could, what would you see? Children tend to imagine that they will be like their parents when they grow up. It's not strange that Brett asked me if he would be on dialysis when he grew up. The question stunned me for a moment. I told him that not all fathers were on dialysis and that there was no reason to believe he would be. I could have said that when he grows up, no one will need to be on dialysis. Medicine will have conquered kidney disease. However, it is better to stick to realities.

Early in my illness, I didn't do much but sit around the house. The children became accustomed to asking Helen for everything. Later, when I was stronger, they still asked her. One day, Scott wanted a ride to some event, but Helen couldn't take him. She had to be someplace else. He kept pleading with her. I was sitting right next to him, but he never once directed a request to me. Finally, I said, "I'll drive you." Everyone in the room suddenly looked at me. I had stunned them. They had adjusted their life-style to my illness, and that had become their norm.

It must be a shock to a youngster to watch a powerful parent figure become helpless and dependent upon a machine for life. That must upset the illusion of immortality that the young have. They are often fearful of the outcome when they go through the usual childhood illnesses. After all, look what happened when Dad got sick.

One morning Brett awoke with severe pain in the right lower abdomen. He was hysterical, and we couldn't figure out why. As we discussed the situation with the pediatrician, he said that he didn't think it was appendicitis. Suddenly, Brett sat up and said, "Whew. I'm glad of that." The pain subsided, and soon he was all right. He had assumed the worst. I'm sure he overreacted because, in the back of his mind, he fears he will end up like me.

Some children may deny dialysis. Scott never says the word. He says, for example, "Are you and Mom going to do it tonight?" The "it" in this case means dialysis, I assume. When I'm on dialysis, he comes into the room only if we ask him to. At other times, he goes there to be alone. There is no question that he evades the issue. My daughters also avoided the dialysis room at first. Gerri simply stayed in her room, and even now rarely visits while I'm on dialysis. Michelle always went to study at a friend's house. She, too, was trying to escape the situation.

The older the child, the more impact the realities of the disease may have. To a four-year-old it may be just another adult thing he doesn't fully understand. The teenage child may realize the life-threatening implications, however. For example, as I discussed college possibilities with Michelle one day, we got around to finances. I was trying to explain that later, if I became unable to work, she could try to get a scholarship. She burst into tears: "I won't take money because my father is dying."

Children can bring humor to the moment. While on dialysis one night, I looked up to see a friend of Brett's staring wide-eyed at me. They were on a tour of the wonders to be found in the house. I was a special attraction. Well, it's better than having him afraid to bring his friends home.

ESRD may reduce you to a child-like dependence, but it may force your children to mature in a hurry. When you can no longer fulfill your roles, someone else must fill them. Children are often thrust into responsibilities beyond their years. Scott, who never touched a kitchen utensil before, learned to prepare his own breakfast, pack his own lunch, and clean up (almost) after himself. Gerri, who couldn't soak a tea bag, learned to prepare dinner.

As my children began to accept dialysis as part of our routine, they began to react more normally. The girls invite friends again, sometimes to stay overnight. Occasionally, I wander down in my shorts on a Saturday morning and am greeted by giggles from strange girls. Scott, who can certainly be heard, if not seen, thunders through the house with his buddies. My dialysis has become for them not much more than an inconvenience, because Helen and I are not as available for school functions, chauffeuring, and the like.

Sometimes it seems they don't realize I'm disabled. One day at breakfast, Gerri was complaining about a back brace she had to wear. I had been wearing leg braces and using a cane for more than a year. She looked at me and said, "Do you know how bad it is to wear a brace and have everyone stare at you? How would you like it?" She just doesn't see me as disabled, I guess.

Brett has also accepted my condition as normal. We were watching TV one night. One of the characters in the show became paralyzed and had to wear braces. Brett turned to Helen and asked, "Has anyone in our family been paralyzed?" Helen looked at me in disbelief. "Your Daddy is paralyzed," she said, somewhat surprised. "No, I mean *really* paralyzed," he answered disdainfully.

5 The Choices

When fluids don't get processed by the kidneys, they stay. There's no place for them to go. As the kidneys get worse, the amount of fluid becomes greater. When I reached this stage—this was about five years after I first learned I had kidney problems—I was becoming like a water-filled balloon, heavy and sagging. Fluid-filled flesh rolls creased my abdomen. My waist had expanded until I had only one suit that would button. I gasped for air after trying to tie my shoes. Though I was always tired, I couldn't sleep at night.

At this time I had a big job to do. I was program chairman for a national medical convention in my hometown. I could barely walk from my hotel room to the elevator. The escalator moved too fast for me to get on. At one point, during a break between sessions, I couldn't endure the fatigue a minute longer. I sank into a plush thick-cushioned bench from which I knew I could never get up by myself. Dozens of people were milling about, and I thought I could easily get help. About 15 minutes later, I was ready, but, without my realizing it, everyone had disappeared.

I was getting desperate. Finally, a man with a convention badge came by. Stranger or not, he was my rescuer. "Can you help me up?" I called. "Sure," he said. Taking my arm, he tugged as I tried to rise. We both fell back into the cushions. Next, I grabbed both his arms and pulled. My tail end rose no more than half an inch. Finally, he grabbed my belt behind my back and pulled. We got up, but I was slowly tilting toward him. About the time he was going to fall over backward, I managed to straighten my knees. We made it . . . after five full minutes!

Somehow I made it through the meeting, but I knew I couldn't go on this way. I said to Helen, "Take me to a doctor. Do anything you want with me. I give up." I got to the hospital so exhausted and defeated that I didn't care what they did to me.

After some time, my nephrologist came to tell me I should have been on dialysis a while ago and that I needed to begin as soon as possible. He told me I could go home with a special diet to restrict my fluids. He emphasized that I had to make a decision—and soon.

When we returned for our appointment, I still hadn't decided. The doctor got right to the point: "You have three choices. You can begin dialysis, you can try for a kidney transplant, or you can die." I didn't answer right away. I thought about the agonies of the past year and about pain and depression. Death, I thought, would be a welcome release from the past and a certain escape from the unknown future. More than that, Helen and the children would be free of the burden I represented. Death was becoming a friend.

Yet, I chose life. To this day, I don't know why and how I came to my decision. Perhaps if my physician had encouraged me to live, I'd have given a different answer. Instead, he emphasized the unpleasant aspects of dialysis, the complications suffered by diabetics in particular, and the limited life expectancy I'd have. I was trembling by the time he finished, and almost choked as I replied, "I have to try. I'm afraid as I've never been afraid in my entire life, but I have to try."

He smiled slightly and nodded in agreement. "I'm glad you said that. You're going to be all right."

Other ESRD patients get less upset about choosing life on dialysis or with a transplant. Perhaps they aren't aware of the implications of the choice. Maybe being a physician gave me just enough knowledge to upset me.

In any event, I chose life with dialysis rather than by kidney transplant. For many, transplantation is an excellent course of action, though there are a lot of problems. The kidneys come from a living person or from a cadaver. Your body considers either as a "foreigner." That is, your body recognizes its own tissues and organs and will try to get rid of anything that doesn't belong—bacteria, a splinter, or a transplanted kidney. The process is known as rejection.

To minimize the chances of rejection, complex tests are performed on you and the new kidney to determine compatibility. The more alike your body and the new kidney are, the less reaction there will be. People who are related are more likely to have similar tissues than are people who are not related. An identical twin is more likely than a distant cousin to match your tissues. A cadaver kidney has even less chance of matching your body. The younger and healthier you are and the younger and healthier the donor, the better the chance that the donor kidney will work.

Your physician has to consider several factors before recommending a transplantation. The good news is that survival figures on transplants are changing as techniques improve. Patients who would not have been accepted for transplant before are now being successfully transplanted. Under development are special treatments for cadaver kidneys so there'll be less chance of rejection.

There are other facts about transplantation that you should consider while coming to a choice for or against it. A successful transplant patient can be very active. To a large measure, he can return to life as he once knew it. He is free of reliance on a machine, his diet is much less stringent, and he is sick less often. The unsuccessful transplant patient's story is different. He may suffer many more complications than a dialysis patient. The medications he must take to prevent kidney rejection can make him susceptible to other infections. Successful or not, transplantation surgery and the post-operative course are far from peaceful. Chapter 7 goes into greater detail about transplants.

Each person must decide for himself whether to take the gamble. One factor that can make it difficult for a patient to decide which way to go is physician bias. The transplant surgeon generally believes that transplantation is the only way to go. The nephrologist, on the other hand, recommends dialysis and says that transplantation is too risky. The patient is caught in the middle.

You might think that I, a physician, chose dialysis for good medical reasons. Actually, I didn't know much about renal failure, transplantation, or dialysis, because, in my practice, I had almost no contact with ESRD patients and had never seen a dialysis machine. There was no relative whom I would ask to donate a kidney. My only brother was older, with a family of his own. In addition, my diabetic condition diminished the chances of success with a kidney transplant, and cadaver kidney failure rates in diabetics were extremely high (they're better now). Further, the diabetic has a tough post-operative period. Basically cautious, I chose dialysis, the lesser of the evils.

Those who go the dialysis route have to choose whether to dialyze at home or at a center. This decision involves many nonmedical factors—practical advantages and disadvantages. Medically, the same thing happens in both places.

Dialysis in a center is relatively effortless. All you have to do is get there and flop on a lounge for a few hours. The staff does all the work. You don't even need to know what it's all about; in fact, some center patients know next to nothing about it. Someone is always right with you in case of an emergency. For some ESRD patients, a visit to the center is a chance to socialize. Though it's more expensive, there has been a financial advantage to going to a center. Medicare covers 80 per cent of allowable costs of both home and in-center dialysis, but didn't allow some of the expenses of dialysis at home. A 1978 modification in the Medicare law tries to deal with this inequity.

However, in-center dialysis means you dialyze at the center's convenience. A few centers schedule dialysis in the evening, though most keep only daytime hours. Some centers have TV, some don't—often the set doesn't work anyway. The air conditioning is for the general comfort (of the staff). You may or may not be allowed to bring food.

Home dialysis offers comforting advantages. It's private. You can scratch where you itch, you can wear what you want. You can turn the TV or stereo on or off, read, write letters, and—perhaps best of all—choose your hours.

Dialysis days are convertible, too. Suppose you usually dialyze on Mondays, Wednesdays, and Fridays, but want to see your daughter in a school play next Wednesday. It's simple to switch to Sunday, Tuesday, Thursday, Saturday, and then back to Monday and your regular schedule.

Home dialysis is great if you like to eat. I've had my best meals (including lasagna, soup, tuna fish salad) on the machine. Virtually all forbidden foods are allowed because, with proper planning, you dialyze them out before you're off the machine. An ESRD diet is tough to take. Dialyzers deserve this indulgence. I'd hate to miss it.

I've talked to patients who take two hours to reach a center, dialyze for four hours, and then travel two hours back. That's a day's work. Home dialysis would be a real time saver for these people. Besides, sometimes you feel rotten when you come off the machine. When that happens, it's a great advantage to be able to plop right into bed.

There are other reasons for choosing home dialysis. It's a lot easier to hold down a job if you can dialyze at your convenience at night. Also, home dialysis is better if you must have as much independence as possible.

You have to realize that a competent and cooperative partner is critical. Few hemodialysis patients can manage at home by themselves. A relative, friend, or paid technician may be your partner. (I'm partial to Helen; she's been my partner in all other things for a long time.) Your partner and you will determine the division of labor. Some patients do almost everything, including inserting their own fistula needles. Some, like me, do very little; I don't have enough control of my hands.

Your partner and you will undergo a training program of three to six weeks. Your partner has to be willing, able, well-adjusted, and psychologically stable. Not everyone can tolerate the blood and the needles. Moreover, spending hours together under trying circumstances puts tremendous pressure on both of you.

When you dialyze at home, you give up a lot of space for equipment and for storage of supplies. Our dialysis setup fills one and one-half rooms. Keeping two months' worth of supplies on hand as protection against late or lost shipments creates a huge pile of boxes. A dialysis lounge (a reclining chair) is necessary, too. Add a few water tanks to deionize and filter the water used in dialysis, and you have a nice array of space consumers. Some people manage to get by with less space, but usually a good part of a room is the minimal requirement.

Though some newer portable machines don't require special plumbing, most models do. It's expensive work. We hired a plumber who tore up our wall, installed the plumbing, and then said that we needed someone else to restore the wall. By the time we were done, we paid more than $200. Under regulations in force at that time, Medicare wouldn't reimburse us for the expense.

Dialysis in the home brings the whole process to household members. If you are at the center, they can ignore the whole business, but if you dialyze at home they're exposed to the whole business. That's fine for some people, not so fine for others.

Most home dialysis patients hate to dialyze in centers. Most center patients wouldn't think of dialyzing at home. I guess it comes down to what your inclinations are and what you get used to.

Kidney Function: Normal and Artificial

6

What your kidneys do is a matter of life and death. Without that function, you die. There's no escaping this fact. That's why it's miraculous that there are so many of us—more than 40,000—who are still living when, according to the rules, we ought to be dead. What is it that kidneys do that's so important? How does dialysis substitute for them? These questions are so complex that even nephrologists can't fully answer them. Since I'm not a nephrologist, I don't pretend to understand the whole complicated system, but I'll explain what I've learned.

Normally, everyone comes equipped with a pair of kidneys: Each weighs about four ounces and is about the size of your fist. Kidneys are purifiers. They remove unwanted chemicals, fluids, and waste materials. As the body's blood passes through the kidneys—18 gallons each hour—tiny filtering systems, or nephrons, remove waste products (urea, for example), excess chemicals (potassium and sodium), excess fluid, poisons, and medicines. The filtered substance is called urine. The urine is collected through a set of tubes (ureters) and stored in the bladder, to be emptied, when convenient, through a discharge canal (urethra). Cleansed blood leaves the kidneys and returns to the body.

The kidneys have a great deal of reserve ability. It's not until a very small portion of kidney function is left that dialysis is needed. Many people go through life quite well with only one kidney, either born that way or because of injury to one kidney.

There are other important functions that kidneys perform. They send a chemical messenger (erythropoietin) to the bone marrow, signaling it to make red blood cells. Damaged kidneys don't produce enough of this hormone. This is one of the factors that make many renal patients anemic.

Damaged kidneys may produce too much of another hormone (renin), which, through a chain of reactions, causes the blood pressure to rise. An excessive amount of renin is one reason why many renal patients have high blood pressure. Sometimes the hypertension is severe enough to require that the damaged kidney be surgically removed.

When the kidneys fail, wastes accumulate, chemicals that should be eliminated build up, fluid collects in the body, and poisons and medicines are not eliminated. Dialysis can take care of these problems somewhat, but doesn't work nearly so well as your normal kidneys. In fact, in a week's time, an artificial kidney removes only 7 or 8 per cent of the wastes that a normal kidney handles.

Healthy kidneys function constantly, keeping the body in a fairly stable condition. In a dialysis patient, however, the wastes and fluids build up and then are suddenly cleansed (in about four hours). They then build up again and are cleansed. It's like stop-and-start driving. It is a tribute to the human body that it can tolerate such changes so well.

Hemodialysis is simply the cleansing of the blood through the use of an artificial kidney. Of course, there has to be some way to get to the circulatory system. A surgically developed shunt or fistula provides the access. In addition, you need an artificial kidney (a dialyzer), through which the blood will pass for cleansing, and a delivery system to supply the dialysate solution to the artificial kidney.

The solution bathes the kidney, and an exchange occurs, across a barrier, between the blood and the dialysate solution. Blood and dialysate do not mix, but chemicals and wastes pass from areas of high concentration within the blood to areas of low concentration within the dialysate. The dialysate drains away, taking the unwanted material with it. The blood returns to the body, cleansed.

Hemodialysis can achieve part of the kidneys' function, but not all. Though it works pretty well to remove wastes, regulate the body chemistry, and control the accumulation of water, you have to cooperate by watching your diet and your fluid intake. For example, when water and salt accumulate, blood pressure rises. An artificial kidney doesn't influence renin production and so is less effective in regulating blood pressure. Since hypertension itself is known to damage kidneys, as well as cause heart disease and strokes, it seems wise to keep your blood pressure down.

Red blood cell production is reduced not only by a lack of erythropoietin, but also by the toxic products of renal failure. By removing the toxic products, an artificial kidney can help manage the anemia. Dialysis doesn't supply erythropoietin, however, and, unfortunately, the chemical cannot be given as a medication.

Kidney patients also often suffer from nutritional and vitamin deficiencies. The artificial kidney will not help here. In fact, dialysis removes some vitamins.

Various machines and dialyzers are used today. Their basic components are: 1) access and return to the circulatory system; 2) a dialyzer or cleanser; 3) a dialysis solution; and 4) a delivery system for the dialysis solution. Modern machines also have monitoring systems that sound an alarm if something goes wrong. In addition, a blood pump circulates the blood faster than your heart can, so more blood passes through the dialyzer. For the usual four-hour session, perhaps 60,000 cc or 60 liters of blood are cleansed.

All dialyzers have some sort of membrane, or barrier, between the dialyzing solution and the blood. It does the work that a normal kidney's nephrons do. The membrane allows small molecules to pass easily, but blocks larger ones. Red blood cells are too big to cross the membrane, but chemicals like potassium and sodium are small and pass readily. Large protein molecules don't pass, but urea does. The ideal membrane would let through all unwanted substances and keep all desirable substances with the blood. There are two problems: The ideal membrane doesn't yet exist, and we don't really know all of the molecules we should get rid of.

Water passes fairly readily back and forth across the membrane, but some factors affect its passage. Each kind of machine controls the pressures on one side of the membrane to force water into the dialysate solution. The water then drains away with the solution.

The dialysate solution contains chemicals in various mixtures that your physician may select. If you dialyze at home, you can get ready-to-use solutions or mix your own. The exchange that occurs between your blood and the dialysate depends, in part, upon the contents of the dialysate solution. Remember, chemicals that can pass across the membrane go from where they are in high concentration to where they are low. This passage stops when the concentrations of a chemical on both sides of the membrane become equal. If you wanted to lower the amount of potassium in your blood, you'd be sure that the concentration of potassium in the dialysate was less than that in the blood. Potassium would then flow into the dialysate. But you wouldn't want to take too much potassium out of the blood. So you make the concentration of potassium in the dialysate high enough to leave the desired amount of potassium in the blood when it reaches the point of stability with the solution.

There are other gadgets (such as heparin pumps and a heating system for your blood and the dialysate). If you're on the machine, or will be, it's good to know how it works. Your physician or the staff at your center will be glad to go into more detail.

There are machines on the market now that are portable. One is so large and heavy that you need a dolly to transport it. It's called portable because its water supply is not permanently connected to the plumbing. A stationary dialyzer gets its water supply from special attachments to plumbing fixtures and drains. The machine mixes the water with concentrated dialysate to produce the solution that flows through the dialyzer. In the portable system, you have to prepare a batch of dialysate solution from powder or concentrate and water before you dialyze. There is no continuous flow of dialysate.

One portable system is called the suitcase kidney (SK). It's really two suitcases. One holds pumps for the dialysate and blood, a polyethylene bag that holds the dialysate solution, and monitoring equipment. The other suitcase holds the disposable materials: tubing, dialysate concentrate, dialyzers. It was designed by Dr. Eli Friedman of New York.

SK dialysis takes the same amount of time as does stationary dialysis. One difference is that the fluid container must be filled at least one more time during the run. The SK has to be plugged in.

Another portable system is run by a 12-volt battery. It's so portable, it can be worn—it's called the wearable artificial kidney (WAK). The patient can disconnect from the tank for up to an hour, but has to get back on it without fail. Dr. Willem Kolff, the Dutch physician who originated dialysis in 1944, designed the WAK.

These two, the SK and the WAK, were designed before the Federal Drug Administration imposed stricter regulations on dialysis machines. But they have been tested and found workable. If they are redesigned to meet Federal regulations, they may soon be on the market.

The advantages of a portable are that there is no installation or tearing up the walls; you can move it to any room in the house, and you can travel with it. Some people—ESRD patients who tested these machines—put them into motor homes, houseboats, or trailers and were free to roam. It'd be nice to have some options left open.

Kidney Transplants

7

Every kidney patient has dreamt of having normal kidney function once again. For many, this dream has come true. Since 1953, more than 24,000 kidney transplants have been performed in the United States. Out of all these transplants, about 45 per cent are still surviving, and some have gone 20 years. Each year, there are 10,000 newly-diagnosed ESRD patients who are considered ideal candidates for transplantation. Only about 3,000 receive kidneys. Why are there not more people receiving transplants?

The number of transplantations is probably rising as we get newer and better medical techniques. Up to now, there have been a lot of factors that prevent transplants.

First, it isn't easy to get the right donor kidney at the right time. There are two sources of kidneys: living donors and cadavers. Some experiments are under way to see whether animal kidneys may be used, but that research is just beginning.

Your body will more readily accept a kidney whose tissues closely resemble your own. Generally, the body recognizes foreign materials and attempts to get rid of them. Someone else's kidney is foreign material, and so your body tries to destroy it. Certain blood cells attack it. So, if you can fool your body into thinking that the grafted kidney is your own, it won't try so hard to reject it. One half of all transplants are rejected within two years. The ideal candidate to provide a kidney is your healthy, legal-aged, identical twin, but not many of us have one. Next on the list is a healthy relative. Third is a cadaver kidney. Since the cadaver probably wouldn't be a relative's, its kidney is less likely to be like yours and more likely to be rejected.

If a relative offers a kidney, that doesn't mean you're home free. Extensive tests need to be made to determine just how much the donor's tissues are like your own.

Besides being sure that kidney tissue matches your body's tissues, the body's reaction to foreign materials can be reduced by drugs. They are called immunosuppressive agents. They decrease the number of cells in the blood that attack foreign materials.

There are many nonmedical problems with getting a kidney. Most transplant patients I know experience a mixture of anxiety and anticipation. Often they have waited and waited for "their kidney" to come along, becoming most anxious on weekends, when the greater number of accidental deaths increases the chances that a kidney will become available. They don't want someone to die, yet hoping for a cadaver kidney has to mean hoping for another's death.

A transplant from a relative is viewed with gratitude diluted by concern. Whom should you ask, and how do you ask him? You could make someone feel guilty if he refuses. Things usually go better when the donor volunteers. In either case, what if the transplant fails, and the donor gave up a kidney for nothing?

What are the risks to a donor? Only 0.1 per cent of

donors die at surgery, so it's a reasonably safe procedure. When one kidney is removed, the other usually enlarges and does the work of two. The donor should feel no different after recovery. From then on, of course, he has only one kidney to lose—as in an auto accident—but the risk is small. Donors go through extensive tests and examinations before they are permitted to undergo surgery, so it's not a snap decision.

While cadaver kidneys have a lower survival rate than kidneys from living donors, that's not why more cadaver kidneys aren't used. It isn't easy to get them. Cadaver kidneys work best if taken from the body while the heart is still beating. That means that the brain has stopped working and the person is truly dead, but that the heart and lungs are still kept going artificially. Under these circumstances, it's hard to decide whether you can take a kidney from the body. You can't ask the patient for permission, and the family is often too upset to make a decision.

In many states, people are asked to sign donor cards and carry them in their wallets. More than 20 states have space on their driver's licenses for the license-holder to note that his or her organs can be used for transplants. If there were more donor kidneys available, not only would that mean there could be more transplants, it would also increase the chances for success. More kidneys would allow for closer matching of donor and patient tissue types.

When you've been offered a kidney and are ready for the transplant, the surgeon attaches the donor kidney's blood vessels to yours and attaches the donor kidney's ureter to your bladder. In a day or so after surgery, you'll be able to eat and get out of bed. You'll need frequent blood tests to make sure the kidney is functioning properly.

Two terrible things can happen after surgery: You can die, or the transplanted kidney may be rejected. Institutions and surgeons claim varying death rates and kidney survival rates. New techniques are changing these numbers. Your doctor has up-to-date information. Even if you once reject a kidney, you can get another. Generally, however, later transplants have less chance of survival than the first.

Your situation following surgery is not without difficulties. Your medical condition will require very close observation, and many problems may evolve. One is that the immunosuppressive agents you have to take to forestall rejection make you prone to infection. These drugs decrease your ability to destroy bacteria.

At one time or another, all transplant patients have a serious bout with infection. The spread of bacteria from the site of an infection is the cause of 80 per cent of the deaths of transplant patients. Infection is most likely to occur at the time of intense treatment against rejection. Infections have to be treated, and the treatment for a serious infection may mean stopping immunosuppressive medications. This greatly increases the possibility of rejection.

You can see that transplantation can occasion severe anxiety. You put so much hope in it, and there are so many risks over which you have no control. The whole episode can be very unpleasant, but if all goes well, you will forget the misery in the joy of having a kidney of your own once again.

For some time you'll need check-ups—more frequent at first, but fewer as your condition improves. These evaluations are essential to spot problems as early as possible so they may be corrected. Among the problems that may arise are high blood pressure, disturbances in the chemical-control systems of your body, difficulties with liver function, the development of tumors, bone problems, cataract formation, and infection. Moreover, the new kidney can develop problems similar to the ones that affected your own kidney.

From the time you try to procure a donor kidney to the time you are living with a transplanted kidney, a number of people can face psychological stress. The physician faces a moral dilemma. He has a patient for whom he wants to provide the best chance at life. He knows that a living, related donor is the best source of a kidney for his patient, but he also knows that he should do no harm as he attempts to cure. He places the donor at risk, which, fortunately, is small; the chances of doing good outweigh the risks of doing harm. But he cannot rationalize away the pain, the anxiety, the cost, and other hardships that the donor faces. He favors getting a kidney from a relative because that's best for the patient. So he won't be accused of putting pressure on a family member to donate a kidney, the physician often has the patient's spouse, parents, or sibling find a donor.

In the case of a cadaver kidney, the physician still faces conflicts. While the physician caring for the renal patient wholeheartedly attempts to obtain a kidney, the physician caring for the potential donor must divide his loyalties. He must safeguard any chance that his dying patient may return to health. By doing this, he may be jeopardizing the chance for a transplant. Not only is he caught between protecting the patient and protecting the kidney, but he must often bear the brunt of communicating to the anxious family the need for the dying patient's kidney. Some hospitals allow a kidney to be taken from a body only if a physician not involved in the transplant declares the person dead.

When the physician enlists the family to find a living, related donor, most often it's the spouse who does the seeking. The spouse, of course, is not a suitable donor, since he or she is not a blood relative. He or she has several advantages over the patient when it comes to asking relatives. The spouse is asking a favor for someone else, whereas the patient would be asking a favor for himself, which can be humiliating. The spouse can exert tremendous pressure on potential donors—it's expected that a spouse should fight for his or her mate. In addition, the spouse is not in the position of asking something of others that he or she wouldn't do. Another relative who is not an acceptable donor can be an effective recruiter for the same reason.

In most instances, it's difficult for the searcher to ask directly. Usually, the process is indirect. The searcher makes relatives aware of the patient's desperate situation and that a kidney transplant is desirable. Then the searcher waits for a volunteer. Subtle or more obvious pressures may be placed on a potential donor. For example, the spouse may say to a relative, "John is getting much worse. He really needs a kidney. Someone in the family just has to help."

The searcher should not be too indirect. In some situations, the pressures can be so subtle and the hints so vague, that potential donors may not realize that they are being asked. If asked more directly, the relative may volunteer.

Some donors make instantaneous decisions and then stick to them. Others need time to review the situation. Relatives who don't want to volunteer often ignore indirect hints or indirect requests. They remain silent, sometimes even run away: A potential donor brother suddenly takes an overseas job; a sister stops visiting and avoids the family. Relatives use other methods to escape the guilt and family displeasure that could follow if they were to refuse directly: "I'd like to donate, but my wife is dead against it," or, "My doctor says I can't."

It could happen that the patient requiring a transplant has done something in the past that makes relatives unwilling to donate. The patient may have been irresponsible, drifting from job to job, borrowing from or living off relatives, always disappointing them. They may feel the patient doesn't deserve a kidney, that he won't reform, that he'd repay generosity with disappointment again. A sibling may have always resented the love and attention that the patient received from their parents. Such a sibling may feel, "He's not going to get my kidney, too!"

A relative may agree to donate a kidney, but then not show for examinations or tests. There may always be a reason for not showing up, but, after a while, a pattern becomes apparent. Instead of saying "No," they simply don't take the needed steps. Some would-be donors have left the hospital on the night before surgery.

Parents are the most likely donors. In our society, mothers, especially, are expected to give everything and anything for their children, but even they may refuse. Adult siblings are the next most likely donors. Adult children rarely donate to their parents, and minors are frequently not permitted by law to donate without special court action.

The so-called "black sheep" of the family are common donors. A sibling who has been drummed out of the family may volunteer, perhaps as a way of getting back into favor.

Most donors, although they may go through a great deal of physical and emotional anguish, end up feeling very good about themselves. Their self-esteem rises because of the selfless act they have done. Particularly if the transplant is successful, the donor is usually elated, and friends and relatives react positively to him or her.

As one might imagine, the patient undergoes a great deal of stress. It's hard for him to ask a relative to volunteer, because of the fear of refusal. Even though he may claim, "I can't expect anyone to give up a kidney," the patient may harbor hostile feelings toward relatives who refuse. Relatives who the patient thought would volunteer may not, and others volunteer who he thought wouldn't.

The patient may view transplantation as the great hope, an escape from unending dialysis. When such expectations are built up, great disappointment may follow. Potential transplant patients must realize that many problems remain even if the transplant is successful. Some physicians take a pessimistic view of transplantation. One such view appeared in an editorial in the Journal of the American Medical Association. In part, it said that "the transplanted kidney can provide only a prolongation of life for the recipient. Hopes that the transplanted kidney will survive are in conflict with the reality that it is probably destined to fail. . . . Imperceptibly, but almost certainly, the transplanted kidney will fail." Protransplant physicians counter with the argument that patients feel better, adapt better, live better, and are better with transplantation. If it's so terrible, they ask, why do patients who have had a transplantation that failed so desperately want another? The controversy goes on, but the patient needs to understand that he won't get back to normal even with a new kidney.

Apart from the anxiety, discomfort, and medical difficulties of the surgery and the postoperative period, the patient who receives a kidney faces many unknowns. The overriding long-term concern is that the new kidney will be rejected. Because of the drugs designed to prevent rejection, the patient may develop unpleasant body changes (acne, facial hair, obesity) that may cause distress. Infection, as noted above, is a constant threat.

There are psychological as well as physiological stages in adapting to a new kidney. At first, the patient may think that the new kidney feels strange, or funny. Gradually, the new kidney is incorporated into the body image until eventually the patient considers it as part of himself. The kidney has gone from "not me" to "me."

Immediately after the transplantation, patients often feel elated, filled with energy, as if they were miraculously healed. Many say that they have been resurrected.

Some recipients—mistakenly, of course—believe that they have taken on attributes of the donor. A brother may fear that he will be lazy like his donor brother. He may feel that, because his donor is lively and cheerful, he will be lively and cheerful, too. A man receiving a woman's kidney may fear feminization.

A patient receiving a cadaver kidney probably won't know anything about the person from whom the kidney came, and so he may fantasize about that person. He may feel that he is younger because the kidney came from a younger person. He may conceive of the donor as a criminal who was shot and killed and fear that he has inherited evil tendencies. Since the donor is unknown, there are no limits to the recipient's imagination.

The patient may think that someone has died in order to give him a kidney. He may feel he has to "make it up" or "pay off a debt" to the donor or to society by becoming an exemplary person.

There are some patients who have grown so accustomed to the sick role, they don't adjust well to a more normal life. Sexual problems hidden by the sick role may surface again, or sexual expectations may rise again after transplantation.

Teenagers seem to have special problems after a transplant. School absences, peer conflicts, problems in sex and dating are common. Physical and psychological changes often seem more than they can handle.

Transplantation may be a very frightening experience for a child because he may not understand what it's all about. A child often relates strongly with his donor, commonly his parent. The parents of the child have to be less protective and to let the child develop.

It should be clear that transplantation is not the land of milk and honey. Most ESRD patients who could be assured of a good chance for a successful transplant would probably elect to have one rather than to dialyze, but the risks and problems that go with it shouldn't be ignored.

8 Peritoneal Dialysis

Peritoneal dialysis is in many ways different from hemodialysis. However, the idea is the same. That is, there is an exchange of chemicals between a dialysate solution and the fluids of the body. At present, peritoneal dialysis is often used for patients who suddenly develop kidney failure because of burns, injuries, or poisonings. Or, if a transplantation is expected very soon, peritoneal dialysis is used to improve a patient's condition for the transplant surgery.

Peritoneal dialysis requires surgery to open the abdominal wall and implant a catheter into the abdominal cavity. Dialysate fluid is washed into and out of the catheter.

Remember that dialysis occurs across a membrane, a thin wall that lets some things pass through and blocks others. In hemodialysis, the membrane is a man-made substance in the machine. In peritoneal dialysis, it's the natural lining of the abdomen. The idea of using this membrane, the peritoneum, isn't new, but it took a while to make it work. In both the artificial kidney and the peritoneum, blood passes on one side of the membrane and dialysate fluid bathes the other side. Materials that you have to get rid of pass out across the membrane from the blood into the dialysate.

An artificial membrane allows some particles to pass more readily than others, and the peritoneal membrane allows others to pass more easily. Your doctor may select or reject peritoneal dialysis because of this difference.

There is a right amount of dialysate that you should use in peritoneal dialysis, and your doctor determines how much—it's usually about two liters or quarts. Your doctor also determines how long it should take for the heated dialysate to enter your body, when to drain it out, and how long that should take. He'll consider your size, your comfort, and the results of your blood tests.

Peritoneal dialysis is well suited for doing at home. It's simple, can be done without a partner, and can be run overnight while you sleep. You can even move around while dialyzing, which you can't easily do on hemodialysis. Peritoneal dialysis is the preferred method for very small children and elderly people. In cases of blood vessel disease or when you repeatedly fail to gain access to your blood vessels, it is a good substitute for hemodialysis. If a patient must dialyze at home, but hemodialysis is not practical, peritoneal dialysis is the common alternative.

The peritoneal method is not without problems. Sometimes the catheter gets blocked or clots. Leaks can break out around the catheter. At times, there may be discomfort. On occasion, the catheter may come out from the abdominal wall. Home patients dialyze four times a week for 10 hours per run. Fortunately, you can get a full night's sleep while it's going on. In-center patients—there are not many—dialyze for 20 hours, twice a week.

Patients on peritoneal dialysis can't travel so readily as hemodialysis patients can. There aren't as many places equipped to care for them. There is some help available, however. American Medical Products Corporation, P.O. Drawer 190, Freehold, N.J. 07728, will help arrange trips and will send supplies to your destination. The booklet "Dialysis World-Wide for the Traveling Patient," obtainable for $1 from the National Association of Patients on Hemodialysis and Transplantation (NAPHT), 505 Northern Boulevard, Great Neck, N.Y. 11021, lists dialysis centers that accept peritoneal dialysis patients.

Peritoneal dialysis can be done by almost anyone at home, and it's cheaper to do it there than to do in-center hemodialysis. Lower cost may make it the more common method of ESRD management.

9

Implanting the Plug

If there was anything that threw me, the physician-patient, for a loss, it was the vascular surgery that's necessary to permit hemodialysis. I had heard about a "little incision" to connect an artery with a vein, but I didn't pay much attention. I guess the other doctors thought I knew what to expect. Well, I didn't.

When I realized that they were going to cut *me*, and do it under local anesthesia, I almost changed my mind about dialysis. They called it a "minor procedure." Minor to the surgeon, maybe, but not to me. I wouldn't even be asleep. "They've got to be kidding," I thought. "There's no way I can go through that!"

Only after the surgery did I learn what the procedure is about. It's necessary because hemodialysis requires an access to the vascular system. To do this, a shunt or a fistula is implanted in the patient.

The shunt is the older method. It's an artificial connection between an artery and a vein. It may be placed in the arm or leg and is external in part. First, an artery and a vein are surgically cut, and a tube is inserted to connect the two. The shunt can be opened to permit the arterial end to connect to one part of the dialysis equipment, and the venous end to another part. Blood runs to the machine from the artery and back into the body through the vein. A shunt can be used to dialyze almost immediately.

Shunts aren't altogether safe, however. Blood clots may develop, the connection may open and cause heavy loss of blood, infections may develop, and the wearer must treat the shunt carefully.

Hemodialysis became more popular when the idea of fistulas came along about 1965. The full name is internal arteriovenous fistula. Skin covers the entire fistula. It's a surgically created artificial connection between an artery and a vein in the arm or the leg. Some fistulas are made by directly connecting the artery to the vein. Occasionally, a graft from a vein in the leg or from a blood vessel of an animal is used to make the connection. Well-constructed artificial fistulas can last for years.

With a fistula, needles that act as vessels are thrust into the venous part to obtain the vascular access and return for the dialysis. The larger the vessel, and the greater the volume and flow of blood in the vessel, the easier and better the dialysis. Blood flows from the artery to the vein because the artery is more muscular and less expandable than the vein and because the pressures in the artery are higher. Over a period of time the vein expands. Since the fistula is under the skin, it's less likely to get infected, clot, bleed, or interfere with life's usual activities. The only disadvantage of a fistula is that about a month must pass before it can be used.

I have both shunt and fistula. I was so sick just before dialysis that the doctors decided on a shunt in my right arm for immediate use, and a fistula in the left arm for later, more permanent use.

Lying in my hospital bed that morning of the surgery, I waited for the this-is-it word. Nothing happened. Hours later, a nurse bounced in and casually said, "The doctor will be a little late getting to you." I wasn't too happy about that. I wanted to end the suspense.

Lunchtime found me still in my bed. To my anxious question the nurse replied, "Oh yes, the doctor will be a little delayed." Afternoon shadows crossed my hospital sheets, and by this time my fingernails were gone.

Eventually, when I'd given up hope of getting any attention, a needle was thrust into my arm and I was being rolled down the hall. I remember heaving a sigh of satisfaction. Little did I realize they had given me Demerol.

It happens that Demerol and I get along like a wino with his bottle. I drifted into a never-never land where I could see, hear, and speak. But not rationally. They tell me I was a riot in the O.R. I called one surgeon a "clean-handed garage mechanic," and I complained to the other, "At least you could introduce yourself before you start cutting."

When my head cleared, I found both arms swathed in inch-thick bandages and wrapped in ice packs. Just as my doctor had said, I could do anything I wanted after surgery—except move my arms. That strongly affects eating, bodily care, and bringing back feeling to numb fingers.

The next day, the ice packs came off. As I began to enjoy the feel of warmth again, I was surrounded by numerous hospital types who cheerfully announced, "We're going to dialysis." As we rumbled down the hall, I thought to myself, "Wait! Is this trip necessary? Let's talk this over." But there was no retreat. From now to forever, three times a week, I had a date with a machine. The impact of that realization was almost overwhelming.

The first encounter presumably went as well as can be expected. I was too weakened to pay much attention. After several runs on dialysis, I was discharged from the hospital, but I doubt that Helen and family were ready to have me home. Remember that I was partially paralyzed in my arms and legs, probably in worse condition than most renal patients. I needed a cane or a walker usually, but neither was helpful now. With my arms wrapped and almost useless, I couldn't walk; and dialysis at first is terribly weakening. I was reduced to a wheelchair.

My shunt required cleansing every time the dressing was changed, but the dressing was not to get wet. Excessive care to keep it dry—avoiding bath water—resulted in a bad case of B.O. For everyone's sake, Helen and I had to develop a technique for my bathing without getting the dressing wet.

Helen would put me in a chair next to the tub, slip a towel under my arms, and lower me into the water. My shunt arm was in Saran Wrap. While I bathed, I'd try to hold up the shunt arm or rest it on the tub's edge. However, the warm water made me sleepy. I'd often be wakened by my arm's splashing into the water. And anyway, even when I stayed awake, I had trouble washing both armpits using only one arm. We struggled this way, with my dialyzing as an out-patient, for about a month. After that, we started dialysis at home.

10

Home Is Where I Can Scratch What Itches

We casually run through our dialysis sessions; after hundreds of them, it's become easy. Still, I marvel that Helen and I ever learned to handle so intricate a system. Right from the beginning, we decided that home dialysis was the only way for us. I was determined to return to work, and Helen wasn't going to have an invalid around the house all day. Fortunately, she's the kind of person who handles major disasters with equilibrium and who copes with adversity. Without a stable partner, home dialysis is bound to fail.

We had to go through a basic training for home dialysis. At that time, I was a mess. I had gained 52 pounds, all of it fluid, and a month of hospital dialysis hadn't taken it off yet. I could stay awake for little more than 30 minutes at a stretch. Sleep was what I did best. What with arms and legs severely weakened by nerve injuries compounding my troubles, I felt altogether useless. Helen had to be the one to do most of the procedures.

On Borrowed Time: Living With Hemodialysis

There were three of us couples in class. Three days a week we dialyzed. We had to get up at 5:00. Helen got me through bath and breakfast, rolled me to the car and into the dialysis center by 6:30. For her part of the course, Helen had to set up the machine, check vital signs (blood pressure, pulse, temperature), record my weight, and insert the fistula needles. She had to prepare the solutions for injection and measure out the drugs. Once a week she drew blood for laboratory tests and ran a hematocrit. Each day she measured clotting times and blood flows. After dialysis, she learned to clean the machine and store the kidney for the next use. After all that, she wheeled me back to the car and then into the house. When she was done putting me to bed, she could start on taking care of the housework.

Two days a week, we sat in class and learned about dialysis, diet, management of emergencies, and how to troubleshoot our machine. You've got to know what to do when air leaks into the machine and into your body. When this happens, you may get confused and babble nonsense. Or what to do when the kidney springs a blood leak, mixing blood and dialysate, and your blood is tied up in the blood-lines and dialyzer. Helen had to learn how to react to low blood pressure so I wouldn't pass out. I had to learn how to correct a fistula needle that had clotted. I'm glad I didn't think about the possibility of an infection getting into my blood stream and spreading to all parts of my body. And I didn't consider the possibility of a power failure while I was dialyzing. I might have given up.

For one month we trained in the center. My weight kept falling. No one knew when I would hit "dry weight," when I would be completely clean of excess fluid. Then one day, as we were dialyzing, I got muscle cramps and a headache. Suddenly, I became pale and sweaty and sick to my stomach. "Hurray, you hit dry weight!" the nurse exclaimed. And so we were declared ready to go on our own.

We rented a dialysis machine and had it placed in what

once was my study—a plumber had already installed the appropriate pipes and drains. The dialysis machine company representative visited our home and checked out the setup. We were ready.

That evening was it—our first time. Helen set everything up. She turned on the water, turned on the machine, and out came a screech. Red lights flashed all over. No water was coming into the machine. We turned every valve we could think of, screamed at each other, kicked the machine, but nothing happened. I don't know what did it, but, just as we were near the height of panic, it worked.

By this time, perspiration beaded Helen's brow. As she held the needle, her hand shook like Jell-O in an earthquake. She was flushed and pressed her lips tightly together. As she advanced toward me, I prayed and closed my eyes. Pop! The needle slid in.

I often wonder, if she had missed that first time, if we had failed that first session, would we have given up? But here we are, years later: We've lived through blood leaks, clogged bloodlines, machine breakdowns, my passing out, more than one power failure, and other adventures. Even after years, after you think you've handled every conceivable problem, something new comes along.

About a year ago, Helen turned on the machine while I was in another room. Suddenly, she screamed for me. Water was spouting from the machine in six directions. It was Sunday evening; try to get a repairman! We called our back-up technician. He had just left for Miami. We called the company representative. He was in Miami. We called the company hotline. "We'll have someone call you right back." He did, thank God! He immediately began asking questions. Then, just like landing a plane by radio instructions, we took the machine apart and repaired it, following his directions over the phone.

You can see that home dialysis is not for the timid. We were reminded of that when the power went out one night.

On Borrowed Time: Living With Hemodialysis

Suddenly, we were sitting in the dark. Of course, I was heparinized—to keep my blood from coagulating—with both fistula needles in place, and the machine wasn't running. Quickly, we mobilized the family: One child got a candle; one looked up the power company's emergency phone number; Helen worked the hand pump to keep the blood circulating; I prayed. Luckily, power was restored in a few minutes, and we went back to dialysis.

One time I passed out cold. We had completed our dialysis run, and I was a bit unsteady, as is usual after a session. My blood pressure was about 110/60, seated. I forced myself to stand and walk to the scale. Apparently, when I stood up, the pressure dropped. My eyes rolled back and my knees buckled. Helen propped my feet up to get more blood to my brain, and I came out of it. Then we had to find a way to get me up off the floor, since, with my muscular weakness, I can't get up without help.

Machinery and I don't get along well. I see machines as enemies that go awry at the moment when they can cause the most trouble. I envision the kidney, filled with my blood, about ready to break down in some new way. We are locked in intimate communion for four hours, three times a week, and during that time I am at its mercy. Not only that, but often throughout the last hour of dialysis, I am miserable. Sometimes, when I get off, I feel as if I had been dragged by horses across a field of tree stumps.

Still, I'd rather feel that way at home than at a center. When I crawl off my lounge, I want to fall into bed, not into my car. I can't say I've learned to love my machine, but I view it now as a servant, not my master. Like my automobile, it's a finicky, demanding servant at times, but it's a useful instrument nevertheless. Perhaps you who dialyze in centers never develop a familiarity with your machines. You drop in, hook up, and leave them behind. I've gotten to feel as if the machine belongs, as if it's part of the furniture.

Home dialysis takes up a lot of space. I can't use my

study for anything except dialysis. The equipment and supplies fill up the space and spill over into another room. One compensation, though, is that you can set up your dialysis unit wherever you want. Some dialyze in their bedrooms. Others use a basement playroom or family room. I have met people who want to be alone and people who want to be where everyone else is.

Many patients look upon dialysis time as lost time. In-center patients are reported to be less likely to make use of the time than are home patients, but I think that's not necessarily so. It's more up to the individual than the place. One in-center patient I know says he's the best-informed man in the city. He reads Newsweek, Time, and U.S. News and World Report cover to cover while dialyzing. Another developed a chess tournament with his neighbor. A teenage patient told me that each time he goes right to sleep and wakes up when his mother takes him off the machine. He even sleeps through having his blood pressure taken! For some people who dialyze on the same schedule in a center, it becomes a social hour.

Most home patients develop their own dialysis routine. Since I spend my days seeing patients, writing research reports, scheduling training programs, and meeting deadlines, I use dialysis to wipe my mind clean. I doze for the first 30 to 60 minutes. Then I eat my supper. By that time, one to one and a half hours are gone. Most of the time I have the TV on, but I'm in some semihypnotic trance. If I don't have a great deal of itching, cramping, or dizziness, the time goes by easily. On occasion, I write letters, read, listen to educational tapes, or play games with Brett. The semireclining position of the lounge is not conducive to concentration. I don't read anything that requires much thought.

Eating in that position, with one hand strapped to the machine, is tricky. Kernels of corn or grains of rice end up in my lap. Bread crumbs find their way into my shirt pocket. I needn't worry about my fluid intake, because I spill half of it.

The position also seems to encourage the collection of gas. I signal the end of dialysis with a giant burp when I sit up.

Some people find dialysis time unbearable. This is more psychological than physical. You can learn ways to change your reactions so you can find dialysis at least tolerable. Some find self-hypnosis a useful tool to make the time pass by more quickly.

In the beginning, Helen was terrified at controlling a machine that held her husband's life. She thrusts two huge bore needles into a vessel that bleeds like an artery if the needles come out. She hooks the tubing up and my blood flows up and into the kidney, turning it deep red. Now the machine has me. All sorts of disasters may occur, blood leaks or air emboli, and all the while I'm anticoagulated.

Home dialysis is more than just a mechanical experience. You and your partner are forced into an intimacy that can become a burden. The two of you put your life in jeopardy every time you dialyze. Physicians are advised not to treat their own families, for good reason: There is too much danger that emotional involvement will cloud judgment. So it is with a husband-wife dialysis team. It's often difficult to separate how you feel about each other from what has to be done to accomplish dialysis.

The husband-wife dialysis partnership can take several forms. One is the "master-slave" relationship: One spouse bosses the other. Some teams are equal partnerships. The nonpatient spouse can be too emotional to do home dialysis successfully: "How can I stick him with a needle when I know how much it hurts?" "I can't force him to limit his fluids. I know I can't." More successful are the spouses who turn off the emotions: "So it hurts, huh? Tough. We've got to do it." These toughies make their partners stick to the rules. Helen is strict. That's probably why we do so well. We always go the full four hours, never three hours and 59 minutes. Those needles go in, ready or not. My moans, groans, and pleadings are met with a stoic response. Helen's a toughie. That's why I'm no longer in a wheelchair and why I've adjusted. She wouldn't let me play sick.

When you're on dialysis, you can't maintain a self-made man, dominating, independent image. You're relatively helpless. Everything you want has to be brought to you. Someone else has to open the window or draw the curtains. Should an emergency arise, you need help. If you have to go to the toilet, too bad. How macho can you be under those circumstances, especially if you're dominated by your wife?

Your partner, too—let's refer to your partner as "she"—has problems. It's difficult for her to express anger and hostility at the situation in which he finds herself directly to you, so she may take it out on others—parents, children, doctors, nurses, organizations. Some spouses, after starting out well, can't take the stresses and eventually quit home dialysis. Others have expressed relief at the ESRD patient's eventual death.

If your partner is angry or irritated, you may be in for a rough dialysis. I don't bring up topics that aggravate Helen. I learned quickly: One night, when I violated that principle, Helen kept missing needle insertions. After five attempts and five failures, we had to quit and try again the next night.

Despite that incident, Helen has become a smooth technician. She has enough confidence to make dinner, do the laundry, or watch TV in another room. But, at the same time, she has become more impersonal about the whole business. I know she at times resents the work and responsibility. At those times, she looks as if she's unconcerned about me and I feel that she's rougher than she needs to be.

While I may sometimes feel I'm a sacrificial lamb, I know that Helen occasionally feels as if she's part of the equipment. When she's covered with blood, or her hands are cracked from formaldehyde, I can read in her eyes that she'd rather be someplace else. The doorbell and dialysis alarm may go off at the same time and cause a frenzy. She may have to stretch out my leg cramps with one hand and adjust pressure gauges with the other. It can be undignified drudgery. But it keeps me alive.

Helen could run away from all these problems. I can't escape dialysis, but she can. Still, each time I suggest that I switch to in-center dialysis, Helen resists. She wants to be there with me.

11

Come on Dialysis With Me

I leave work early. Not that I want to hurry to what awaits me, but I know that the earlier I begin, the sooner it's over. After all these dialyses, you'd think I'd be used to it. But I still have a voice inside me that says, "Not tonight. Why does it have to be tonight?" Monotony is my worst enemy. There is no end in sight. I will dialyze till I die.

I walk out into the sunshine. It's too glorious a day to lie body to body with my machine. But I've got to get home to my fate. The car is superheated from the Georgia sun. Although it's only April, in the car, it's summer. Once I get rolling, I can't adjust the windows or fix the radio unless I stop, because one hand is on the gas/brake lever and the other on the steering wheel. I pray that I don't itch or sneeze. I haven't decided which is worse.

As I weave through the twisting roads toward home, I think about my intestinal tract. It has a mind of its own, and moves when it wants to. Unless I empty it before I go on the

machine, I may end up with a big bellyache and not be able
to relieve it for four hours. The thought preys on my mind
and probably will make me get an urge while strapped to the
machine. When I first began dialysis, I alternated between
severe constipation and severe diarrhea. Once I was caught
on the machine with diarrhea that I had to hold for four
hours. I've never forgotten.

Home is on the top of a hill. I can't walk up, so I have to
park close to the house. Once, when I first became ill, I woke
up at about 6:00 A.M. and went for a walk outside without
waking anyone. I was all right in the level carport, but after
10 feet of slope, I tripped. I'd have rolled down the entire hill
if I hadn't grabbed the gaslight post. There I lay in the wet
grass on my back like an overturned turtle. I didn't want to
wake the neighbors, so I called not too loudly for help. When
no one came, I started banging the gaslight post with my
cane. Finally, a neighbor saw me and called Helen, who
came and pulled me up on my feet. Since then, I've tried no
early morning walks.

Each day, as soon as I enter the house, I habitually go
directly to the refrigerator. I can't eat much, of course; it's
usually just a "take a look and find nothing" affair. Except
on nights when I dialyze. That's when I revisit gastronomic
delights such as corned beef, salami, ice cream, tuna fish, hot
dogs, and the like. My children call it "pigging out." One
reason I do this is that without additional salt, I cramp on
dialysis so badly that I have to reduce the transmembrane
pressure, and then I don't take off enough fluid. By eating
salted foods I avoid the cramping and take off more fluid.
Also, I feel better after dialysis. The second reason I "pig
out" is psychological. On dialysis night I know I can mix a
reward with my misery.

Finally, I can't avoid it. I've gone to the bathroom,
brushed my teeth, and stalled as best I can. I enter the
dialysis room feeling like a virgin sacrifice to the Cordis-Dow
machine. The machine hums, its green light says, "Go, go,

go." The thermometer in my mouth, I climb onto the scale, which will tattle if I dared drink an extra few ounces since last dialysis. "That can't be right!" is my usual protest. "The scale's wrong. I was careful. I *couldn't* have gained that much." I've conveniently forgotten the Jell-O or the extra fruit serving or the half-yogurt I snitched.

Then I'm on the lounge. Its smooth naugahyde finish is cool now, but in a couple hours it will make my shirt stick to my sweaty back. Helen has set up the machine and has laid out all the paraphernalia. It has the feel of an operating room. I tilt the lounge back and wait.

Helen cleans the fistula site on my left arm with betadine pledgets. The sensation of the pledgets rubbing across my fistula chills my spine. The machine whirs. The dials say it's ready to go. The alcohol feels cold and wet as Helen washes off the yellow betadine.

I close my eyes. "Forever. You'll do this forever. There is no escape," the voice inside cries. Momentarily, I'm depressed. I want to cry, "Why me?" But I clench my teeth.

I feel the tourniquet tighten. Most of the time, the huge bore needle slides in and there is no pain. But sometimes the pain is overwhelming, not just as the needle pierces the skin—that's sharp and stinging—but, sometimes, as it pierces the vessel, there is a deep aching that lasts for 10 or 15 minutes. It can happen, though it's rare, that the needle goes through the vessel and out the other side. Then, as blood pours into the surrounding tissue, the pain builds. Sometimes Helen misses, and we end up with four or five needle sticks instead of the usual two. Each time the tourniquet goes on, the agony builds. Knowing all this, I cringe each time Helen inserts the needle. The puncture may be painless and the insertion perfect, yet the anticipation of pain is almost as bad as pain itself.

Now the deep crimson rises in the arterial blood line, and soon stains the dialyzer. The redness slowly fills the kidney and then enters venous line. I never think about the line breaking or the connections coming apart. I know I could bleed to death very rapidly, but I simply ignore this possibility. I couldn't tolerate it.

Now a chill comes over me as the blood returns to my body a few degrees colder. Helen covers me with a blanket, and I position my fistula arm against a pillow so it won't fall as I nap. Whether it's a reaction to the emotional trauma, a way of escape, or just fatigue, I almost always nap right after I go on dialysis. Helen awakens me with dinner.

I eat the meal with my one free hand. The meat is cut into bite-sized pieces, the canned fruit into spoon-sized chunks. Rarely do I drink anything, except the liquid from the canned fruit. Macaroni falls into my lap. Crumbs trickle into my shirt. But I eat. It passes the time. Sometimes it even tastes good, since I can eat forbidden foods.

Every once in a while, the machine blinks warning lights and screeches alarms. Blood leak, arterial pressure, conductivity gauge—they all may flash. If the arterial needle is up against the wall of the fistula vessel, I can feel it sucking against the fistula, stinging and burning. Helen adjusts it, and I close my eyes again, making it all go away.

Two hours to go. I feel light-headed, a little woozy. I'd like to drift into space, but a headache begins to pound. I can feel the skin shrink as fluid is sucked away.

My back itches, and the itch spreads. I shift position and set off an alarm. "Got to lie still," I tell myself. "It'll pass." But, it doesn't. Helen rubs powder on my back, and the itching eases. I've begun to perspire, only lightly, but it's making me uncomfortable. I take off the blanket, and cool air chills me as the perspiration evaporates.

A cramp begins in my left leg. I move it, and the cramp eases, but I know it'll come back. One hour to go. I feel a little nauseated, my legs are feeling tight. A cramp clutches my hands. My God, they hurt. There, it's gone. Now it's in my leg again. I cry for help. Helen stretches my foot, and the cramp eases. She lowers the transmembrane pressure, and the cramps ease off. I eat something salty and I feel better.

Then I feel faint. My head hurts, my gut begins to churn; maybe I'm going to throw up. Cramps squeeze my legs and arms. Helen can't grab all of them, so she calls for help. Sometimes it takes one son, sometimes two to stretch my limbs. Straighten the knee, and the muscles that bend it loosen, but the muscles that straighten it tighten up. Bend my knee, and the opposite happens. "My God," I cry. "How much longer?" Helen tilts the lounge, so that my legs are above the level of my head. She adjusts the machine.

Now it's time to come off. Helen tries to remove the fistula needle, but I'm cramping again. "You'll just have to cramp until I get this out," she cries. The needle is out, and I'm pressing on the cotton pad to stop the bleeding. My leg is tearing me apart. Finally, she grabs it and stretches my heel cord. The cramp eases. Now the last of the blood in the machine returns to my body. My dizziness lessens, my headache eases. I hold both the arterial and venous puncture sites, while Helen cleans the machine. She wraps the wound areas and checks my vital signs. I want to sleep more than anything else. First, I have to check my weight. Then I stagger into the bedroom.

My head swims, and I lose my balance as I approach my bed. The headache is back, but it's dulled by drowsiness. The pillow can't muffle the pounding in my skull. I stretch my body, and my legs spasm with cramps. I sit up, place my foot flat on the floor, and push my knee down. The heel cord gradually relaxes.

If each dialysis were this bad, I couldn't live this way. Some are worse, but most are better. Someone who has never gone through dialysis can't fully understand what it's like, but perhaps I've helped you walk in my shoes for a while. Maybe you felt what I feel.

12 Dialysis Diet

All ESRD patients at some time complain about their diet. I call mine the "blah diet": If I can taste it, I can't eat it. Of course, mine is especially restricted because of my diabetes.

Dieticians are generally nice people. Some of my best friends are dieticians. But I've learned to cringe when they mention sodium, potassium, phosphates, and calories.

Really, I do understand that, since my kidneys don't work, my internal chemical balance is messed up. I know that my body doesn't eliminate potassium properly, and, when potassium levels get too high, my heart may stop . . . suddenly. I know that chocolate cake with chocolate icing is loaded with potassium. I know, but there are moments when I don't care. There are moments when I'd almost kill to taste that creamy, fudgy, chocolaty, yummy stuff on my tongue.

When my salt-free butter melts over my salt-free vegetables lying next to my salt-free four-ounce steak, my hand trembles toward the salt shaker. Sometimes it's will power and sometimes a smack on my hand from Helen that keeps me from devil salt.

The trouble with a diet is that it's there every day. Everything you put in your mouth reminds you of your afflictions. Snack time goody machines display chocolate, nuts, potato chips, and cheese in row after row. There isn't much that comes out of a machine that you can eat. The same may be said about cans and boxes. Read the labels. They list the ingredients according to relative quantity in the product. If salt is third on the list, then it's the third most plentiful item among the ingredients. Even frozen foods may have salt added.

Be careful of hidden salt. Tenderizers often contain monosodium glutamate. Some diet soft drinks have salt. Substitute-salt preparations frequently exchange potassium for sodium. You can almost assume, unless the package specifically says so, that any box or can contains sodium and/or potassium.

I remember my first salt-free canned food. One day, I purchased at a health food store a single-serving can of salt-free soup. I figured it would fit my fluid allotment and I wanted to taste soup again. I heated it up, lovingly ladled it into a dish, and with great anticipation, tasted it. Hot water has more flavor, particularly if it's rusty. Salt-free tuna looks real, smells real, but tastes like clay. I don't like clay.

For a short period of time in the hospital, the dietician put me on a diet with breads, rolls, and cookies made with low-protein wheat starch. The bread came carefully wrapped in tin foil. It smelled pretty good. It looked like French bread. It tasted like crisp cardboard. The rolls were a little better, but they crumbled. I've heard that the cookies can be very tasty, but no one told the hospital baker how to make them that way.

"Water, water everywhere, but not a drop to drink"—a line truer for no one more than a renal patient. You know you are thirsty when you sneak a drink from the shower as

you wash. You know you are thirsty when you lick the drinking cup after taking your morning pills. You're always
thirsty. You turn on the TV and see someone gulping down
an iced tea or a Mr. Sweetheart soda pop. You go to the ball
game and step over the empty beer cups. You go to a restaurant, and they stick a glass of water in your face.

It's not just what you drink that is the problem. Almost
everything you eat has fluid. How about a bowl of Jell-O?
No, you don't. If it is liquid at room temperature, it's a drink.
Sauces and gravies—even without salt—are fluids. An apple
perhaps? At least 85 per cent of it is fluid. So there you have
it, you are surrounded by fluid.

I won't describe the renal patient's diet in terms of
grams and milliequivalents. I'll tell you instead how I live on
a renal diet. My fluid limit is 16 ounces per day. I separate
my beverages into four four-ounce servings: one at breakfast,
one at afternoon coffee break, and one after dinner. That
leaves four ounces to splurge on whenever I wish. When
thirst overcomes me, I rinse my mouth with ice-cold water.
Ice chips can satisfy with little fluid intake. I push water
away if it is offered in a restaurant. When my weight jumps
five or six pounds, I have been tippling a mouthful here and
a mouthful there, or I've been eating too many fruits, vegetables, and salads that contain a lot of fluid. I often find myself
spooning up the juice from my portion of canned fruit, even
though I know it's fluid.

If you're careful between dialysis runs, and your lab
work stays good, you may be able to do what I do. I can't stay
away from flavor forever. So, just before or early in dialysis,
I treat myself with spaghetti, or franks and beans, or ham
and cheese, or tuna, or anything I can't have the rest of the
time. Potatoes, on dialysis, don't lose their flavor very much,
but they do lose their potassium. I've heard of one man who
admits to eating banana sandwiches while on the machine.

Some centers don't allow patients to bring in food;
some frown on "off-limit" foods on dialysis. I think that

anything that makes people enjoy their dialysis sessions is a good idea. People are more likely to stick to a diet if they know that on occasion they can break away. By letting them splurge when it's least likely to cause damage, you are likely to prevent splurging at a more dangerous moment. Some doctors agree with me and some don't. But not many doctors have to stick to diets for years. They may know what is medically indicated, but often they don't recognize what is humanly reasonable.

You can rearrange a renal diet to fit in special events. If you adjust your eating plan over a period from one dialysis to the next, you can be more liberal at a given meal than you might expect. Suppose you are going to dinner on Saturday night—you can almost taste the beef Wellington, the wine, the salty butter on hot bread. Your conscience protests. But wait! If you carefully limit your salt, potassium, protein, and fluid from the time of your last dialysis, you can splurge on Saturday night. What matters in a renal diet is the *total* intake between dialyses. Of course, if you've had a large amount of protein you may want to cover the phosphates with a little extra aluminum hydroxide. Also, be aware that a lot of salt at one sitting will make you thirsty. You can adjust your eating to permit various kinds of splurges. One person I know has a banana split (better known in our circles as a potassium deluxe) on his birthday. One day just before dialysis I even ate a pickle!

I've found that forbidden foods don't taste so good as I had remembered them or dreamed them to taste. Chocolate ice cream is as forbidden for me as anything I can imagine. But, one time, by carefully rearranging my life, I saved up enough room for it in my diet. There it was, on the top of a crunchy cone. The ice cream glistened, not yet melted enough to drip down the cone. I tingled with anticipation. "Pop," went my reverie. It tasted only slightly chocolaty, only mildly sweet, and only faintly creamy. It wasn't very good. Since then, I've decided that if I'm going to work for something special, it's going to be worth it. If I eat cherry cheesecake, it's not going to be a cheap imitation. If it's a hot dog, it'll be the best hot dog I can get. At least then it'll be worth the suffering I have to go through to make room for it.

I have a diabetic diet to worry about, too. I have to watch calories along with everything else. When I first became diabetic, I used to joke that I'd end up on sugar-free baby food. Close. I can't eat baby food. It's too salty!

There are nutritional benefits to the renal diet. You probably have never eaten so wisely. You've been saved from trash foods and empty calories. Helen and I used to beg, cajole, and browbeat our kids about eating junk. I commonly referred to it as "that crap." One day when he was about three, Mommy took Brett to the grocery. He kept tugging at her skirt, trying to ask for something. "Speak louder," she called down to him. Just as he yelled back, the people nearby became quiet. "Can we buy some crap?" he screamed. Every head turned to watch Helen turn red and turn away. There isn't so much "crap" around our house as before.

In the beginning, mealtime was the center of my day. I made sure I received every milligram of food to which I was entitled. I also became upset if my morsels weren't prepared exactly right. If I was limited to a four-ounce steak, it wasn't going to be overcooked. If I was going to eat a sandwich with only a piece of fruit for my fluid, the bread better not be stale and dry. Any piece of fruit had to be perfect, or I would rage about wasting my calories and fluid. I've gotten better about that, but I still get finicky at times.

One of my pet complaints is getting a cold baked potato in a restaurant. After all the planning and skimping I go through to afford that potato, I want it hot. Rather than suffer frustration, I send it back, usually with success.

You need to consult food lists carefully. If you have lists from more than one source, you'll find discrepancies. One item may be under "low potassium" in one list and under "moderate potassium" in another list. Even dieticians can't answer tricky questions sometimes. By scrutinizing lists, you may find that you can eat foods you may have presumed you couldn't. For example, oranges are usually limited or off your list completely. Tangerines are very close in flavor and texture, but low in potassium. I find the substitution quite satisfying. Raw peaches are high in potassium, but canned peaches are low; at least you can have peaches.

When you stick to your diet and control your fluids, you really do feel better. I'm convinced of that. Still, I dissolve at the sight of a pastrami on rye with mustard and a pickle.

13

Husbands, Wives, and Strangers

Chronic illness, as nothing else, tests the mettle of a marriage or other relationship. From personality changes to financial stresses, ESRD bends and twists almost every facet of married life. So both you and your spouse are really different people now. You may feel that your spouse is a stranger, even if you've been married for 20 years.

All living creatures constantly undergo change. We are influenced by personal experiences, by what we read, what we see, our successes, and our failures. Illness, especially chronic illness, is an experience that can alter our outlook, our self-image, and our expectations.

We have mentioned roles several times, and we have pointed out that illness changes them. Because of roles, we all develop expectations for ourselves and for other people. Over the years, husband and wife each learns how the other reacts to certain situations, what each can and can't do. Along comes ESRD, and all our expectations about our partner change, because the patient is now a different person and the spouse must now be a different person. It is the ability to regain a new working arrangement between partners that determines whether a marriage will survive. Things cannot be again what they were before ESRD. You can't expect to return to the "good old days."

I took part in a study to determine in which areas of life ESRD patients were most dissatisfied. We asked about medical health, ability to care for oneself, about sex, finances, family life, social life, opinion of oneself, ability to get around, ability to use one's hands, and about spare-time activities and work. We found that the most common areas of dissatisfaction were finances and sex. That's not surprising, since the general population probably would indicate the same areas of discontent. Most of the 16 per cent of patients who were employed were satisfied about their work situations. The study showed mixed reactions to family and social life, some patients were unhappy and some contented.

Important husband-wife relationships revolve around money. Think about the arguments you and your spouse have had. How many were related to money or an issue that could have been solved if you had money to burn? "We ought to go to the beach for our vacation." "No, I want to go to the mountains!" If you had enough money you could go to both. "It's time to get a new refrigerator." "But I need a new car." Buy both; all you need is money. It may not make you happy, but it makes misery easier to live with.

ESRD puts patients and their families in difficult financial situations. It increases normal financial stresses. But beyond the dollar itself, there are roles that spouses play in regard to money. These roles get mixed up with masculinity and femininity, strength and weakness, and a place in the family structure.

When I was very ill, Helen had to handle our finances. With all she had been through, taking care of me, tolerating my new irritable behavior, and taking care of the family, you'd think that managing the finances wouldn't have been an issue. But Helen has always preferred the old-fashioned role: Husbands provide, protect, and care for wives. That includes finances. She resented assuming the financial role more than anything else. Going to the movies, she would drive—later, I found this irritated her also—but, when I would let her pay at the box office, she wouldn't tolerate it. That simply changed our roles too much.

Control of money often implies control of the family. Does the source of income also determine the distribution of the money? For example, does the wife have to ask the husband for grocery money or shopping money? Or does the husband have to request poker money? Money control means power to many people. Loss of money control means a loss of power, prestige, or status.

Children know whom to go to in order to get what they want. "May I sleep over at Billy's house?" Mom may be the decision maker on that issue. "May I use the car?" "Go ask your father." "I'm going to throw up!" "Quick, get your mother!" The same is true of money. Children learn to get their allowance from the allowance distributor, to get money for clothes, books, or other items from the person most likely to provide money. When roles change with ESRD, the patient is well aware that the children sense the difference. His position in the family structure has changed. Money, again, is not simply a matter of dollars.

With every toothpaste commercial, every clothing ad, and even automobile commercials pushing sex, it is no wonder that we have exaggerated expectations about it. Articles and books tell you how to do it, what to expect (starbursts and fireworks), and how often you are supposed to be active.

Sex is sold as the act of sexual intercourse, and not the relationship between a man and a woman. But sexuality is many things. It's expressed in the way we dress, the way we walk, the way we talk, and the work we do. The younger generation is less male-female role oriented, but my generation has very strong ideas of what a man is and does and what a woman is and does. I still think "female" when I see long hair. I still think "male" when I picture an airplane pilot. Jeans and boots I've grown accustomed to as unisex, but dresses are still only for women. If you tell me someone chews tobacco, I don't picture Miss America!

Sex includes how a man and a woman interrelate. It's partially the act of intercourse, but, in some cases, it includes dominance and dependency roles, breadwinner images, and other areas. In the most obvious sense, however, problems do show up in the bedroom.

Don't lose sight of several important considerations concerning sex. First, a satisfactory sexual life is based on what makes both partners happy. If you never have intercourse and both of you are content with a caring relationship, why be upset if the rest of the world is different? On the other hand, if one partner is content and the other is not, you've got a problem no matter how closely your bedroom activity matches the national average.

Second, you can't base your standards for sexual contentment on the media. Movies, books, and commercials overdramatize sex as they overdramatize everything else.

Third, there are many roads to sexual satisfaction. What each couple does, so long as both partners are happy with it, should not be subject to the approval of others. After all, what they do in their bedroom really is their business.

It is a rare ESRD family that does not have a sexual problem. Both men and women note a decreased desire for sex and a decrease in sexual activity. Often, men become impotent. The problem may be due to a deterioration in self-image. The ESRD patient is often thought of as "sick," and sick people don't engage in sex! Muscles atrophy, and the body changes. As a result, the patient may be less attractive, both in his or her own eyes and to the spouse. Fatigue may play a part: Especially after nighttime dialysis, the patient may be too tired to think about sex, and so the opportunities for sex decrease. Fear of failure to perform satisfactorily may keep the patient from trying. One partner may be punishing the other by withholding sex. Some patients fear bodily injury during sex.

Many couples don't communicate with each other about their sexual dissatisfaction. Instead of discussing sex, they fight over all sorts of other things. Instead of complaining that she is sexually frustrated, a wife may launch a tirade upon her husband for leaving his shoes in the middle of the floor. To avoid intercourse, a husband may eat crackers in bed to aggravate his wife. When she's aggravated, she's not "in the mood." He makes the lack of intercourse her fault, not his. His fear of failure to perform remains hidden.

Not satisfied sexually, the partners avoid displays of affection for each other. After all, why bring up a painful problem? The children very quickly pick up the lack of affection between parents. Often, they fear a divorce, since divorce is alarmingly common among families of their peers.

Sometimes one spouse is not aware that the other is unhappy about sex. If you think you have a problem, there are several sources of help to turn to. The first people who may help are the nurse, the social worker, and the nephrologist in your center. Often, they can settle common problems in a brief discussion. Psychologists, family counselors, sex counselors, and psychiatrists are the people to see for help with more complex problems. Many clergy are now trained in sex counseling. Help is available, but you need to let someone know you need it.

Husband-wife problems may begin even before the diagnosis of renal disease is made. As the kidneys deteriorate, the patient may become irritable, forgetful, confused, withdrawn, and show other intellectual and emotional changes. The patient may not understand what is happening and may become depressed or flare out in anger and frustration. Unfortunately, the most convenient targets of these flare-outs are the members of the household. The spouse doesn't understand what is going on either, and considerable tension can develop in the marriage. It's almost a relief to learn the cause for all these changes. But at the same time, the diagnosis and the fear of the coming renal failure create their own tensions, depressions, and frustrations.

As the patient becomes more dependent on others, he may feel guilty that he can't hold up his end. Anger may alternate with the guilt, but, because it's not socially acceptable to be angry at the person who is helping you, the anger is often not expressed. But anger and hostility spill out. I remember one time when I startled and upset Helen with my anger. I was able to walk only on level ground and I had to walk daily to build my strength. Because our house is on a hill, Helen had to drive me down to where I could walk and then drive me back up the hill. She wasn't always ready to take me when I was ready to go. I'd get frustrated and humiliated because I felt I had to beg her to take me. One evening, after I asked her several times, she finally took me down the hill. When we got there, my rage spilled over. "I hate you," I hissed. "I can't wait 'til I can go by myself, instead of having to wait for you!" It wasn't the first time I had let my frustrations out on her, but it was the most direct hostility I had displayed. I was fortunate that she knew it was my illness speaking, not me.

Someone who has always been dependent may find in illness an excuse to increase dependency. Now it's justifiable to be waited on, babied, cared for. This dependency carries over nicely into dialysis, which requires a degree of dependency, anyway. The dependent role may spill over into sex. Particularly in the male, who is expected to take a more active sexual role, dependency may contribute to impotency.

Families that successfully coped with problems before ESRD are better able to cope with the problems of ESRD. People who are able to accept help adapt more easily to dialysis. The husband who cannot bear to receive help from his wife, yet can't help himself, is in a frustrating situation.

80

Flexible people, who don't follow rigid rules or codes of behavior, are better able to cope. The dialysis patient who feels that a husband must do this and a wife must do that will run into many situations that don't fit his pattern.

Success in coping seems to be related to socioeconomic status. It's easier to be rich and sick than it is to be poor and sick. The rich can buy services they can no longer perform; a yardman does the lawn, a maid does the housework.

In our society, the healthy are expected to "give" to the unhealthy. You give your seat on a bus to a person on crutches, for example. The healthy spouse is expected to yield to the needs of the ESRD spouse. Helen and I still have conflicts. I try to keep my dialysis schedule from interfering with the family's activities as much as possible. Yet, I have to plan dialysis around professional activities that I can't miss. Inevitably, some of these clash with Helen's activities. Also, some social affairs important to her aren't important to me. When activities for one or the other of us are scheduled for three or four nights in a row, someone has to give in, and usually it's Helen.

The husband and wife relationship works best when it is not all one-sided. Each must be willing to give, each must need the other, the pair must be interdependent. I need Helen very badly, but she still needs me. If I ever reach the point at which I no longer contribute, but only take, I don't know what I'll do.

The spouse of the dialysis patient must have a high tolerance for stress and can't disintegrate with every crisis. The spouse can't successfully be a dependent person because responsibility goes with being married to a renal patient.

These stresses and strains are even greater for couples who dialyze at home. Unrelieved togetherness in situations fraught with potential danger and loaded with psychological pressure place the home dialysis couple in constant potential conflict. The issues of dependency, male-female roles, and dominance come to a peak. Dialysis cannot be something that occurs "over there." It is constantly made obvious to the whole family. It can't be ignored.

Parents become particularly involved in the problems of dialysis. Imagine a son or daughter on dialysis, or married to a dialysis patient. How detached could you be? Of course, mothers who perform home dialysis for their children are directly involved. But parents of adult patients often can't avoid facing the significance of ESRD.

When I first became ill, my mother couldn't visit me because she was ill herself. Later, she always found excuses to stay home. Finally, we convinced her to come. On the second night of her stay I had to dialyze. She sat through the entire dialysis without flinching. I asked her if, really, she hadn't been afraid to visit. She admitted that she was torn between her desire to be with her son and the fear of what she would find. But once she made up her mind to come, she was determined not to show her emotions. "After all," she said, "if you and Helen can go through this, so can I."

A supportive family is the key ingredient in rehabilitation for any disabled individual. A patient who feels still loved, respected, and worthwhile, has a good chance of rebuilding his life.

14 Going Back to Work

In the beginning of my illness, despite my reliance on a wheelchair, I insisted on returning to work. Helen would pull me out of bed, dress me, and drive me to the office. On days when I was too sick to see patients, I answered mail, read medical journals, and went home a few hours later. In view of all the obstacles, why did I bother?

Money was certainly a factor. Disability benefits were good, but work income was better. Still, dollars weren't the big reason. I wanted to keep up as much of my previous routine as possible, because work was part of my identity. My mind told me I'd no longer be a man if I stopped work. Work also provides a great deal of my social life, for my workday is filled with many different people and events. Without them, life would be so much narrower.

Obviously, it's hard for me to understand why so few ESRD patients return to work. The problem has intrigued me enough to look into it some more.

On Borrowed Time: Living With Hemodialysis

The first important concept I found is that work does not mean paid employment only. Anything you do that's useful, productive, or meaningful is work, too, even without wages. This applies to the wife-mother-homemaker who generally labors longer than do other kinds of employees; the student who puts all his effort into learning; the volunteers who perform all kinds of tasks for hospitals and charitable, religious, and political organizations. There are many ways to work without pay.

However, not all ESRD patients are unhappy about not working. A study conducted some time ago revealed that only 16 per cent of an ESRD-patient group had returned to the same or to a higher level of employment, housework, or student activity they had before becoming ill. The others, 84 per cent, did not claim that medical complications or fatigue kept them from work. Of these, 51 per cent said they were satisfied with their situations; only 16 per cent were not, while the rest were undecided. I find this discouraging.

Unfortunately, some people who want to work are trapped by circumstances. If a manual laborer with little education develops ESRD and can't return to his usual work, what are his chances of finding other employment?

What about in-center dialysis patients in general? They usually have treatment during the day, three times a week. That makes dialysis, and the time needed to travel to and from the center, practically a full-time occupation. Of course, in-center patients who can dialyze at night are better able to return to their jobs.

Home dialysis patients' work opportunities also are limited. Besides the hours dialyzing, it takes time to set up the equipment, to clean up, and to recover afterward.

Another fly in the ointment: Employers are often reluctant to hire ESRD patients. Even when company management is willing, union regulations may intervene. Or supervisors and co-workers are suspicious of the patient's ability to do his fair share.

In addition, families may contribute to patient failure to resume normal-as-possible living patterns. By overprotecting, relatives may "kill with kindness." Just like giving a child all the sweets he wants, the results could prove disastrous, physically and emotionally. If the patient's needs are quickly anticipated and met, all he has to do is be sick. "Why work?" he may ask.

Similarly, families that push too hard also contribute to patient failure. If more is expected of the patient than he can do, he'll fail. If he fails often enough, he'll stop trying. Balancing patient capacities with the job is absolutely essential.

Moreover, ESRD patients sometimes find it's not financially rewarding to work. Most are on Medicare, which pays about 80 per cent of the medical bills. The remaining 20 per cent is paid by the patient or insurance (for center patients, it may be waived if insurance doesn't cover it). Medicaid picks up the tab for some. Let's add Social Security disability income (about $3,000 per year) plus any clauses in life insurance, car loan, and home mortgage contracts that cancel payments because of disability (another $3,000, at least). Here's a tidy sum—available by not working.

Recent research figures indicate that about two thirds of ESRD patients who return to work gross less than $10,000 a year. Considering assorted taxes and other items taken from the paychecks, these patients are likely to profit by staying at home.

Nevertheless, if you want to work, there is help. Each state has a vocational rehabilitation agency with offices located in various parts of the state. Counselors advise handicapped people, including ESRD patients, who have trouble finding employment. Evaluations, treatment, transportation, training, job placement, and even tools and equipment when appropriate, are provided by the agencies. They have no system for finding you, however. You must call them.

Of far-reaching consequence is the Rehabilitation Act of 1973. It states that every employer awarded a Federal contract of more than $2,500 must take "affirmative action" to hire handicapped people. Their job assignments, promotions, training, transfers, and so on are also covered. The Act requires not only management but labor unions as well to make accommodations for the handicapped.

In essence, if you are competing with nonhandicapped job seekers, equally qualified, you should have the advantage. The ESRD patient is surely more acceptable for certain occupations than are paraplegics or people with coronary-circulatory disease.

For a guide to the Rehabilitation Act of 1973, write to the President's Committee on Employment of the Handicapped, Washington, D.C. 20210.

Public Law 95-292 makes End Stage Renal Disease Program changes that may enable more home-dialysis patients to return to work. The law eliminates the three-month waiting period now in effect before Medicare benefits for home dialysis are paid. The law also requires the government to pick up more of the costs of home dialysis, and provide for some professional assistance in the home.

Social Security law contains a helpful provision, too. It permits people to return to work, for nine to 12 months, without losing disability benefits. This trial-basis period gives you a risk-free chance to decide whether employment is profitable for you—fiscally and physically.

What it all boils down to is this: If you're able, how badly do you need and want to work? Each of us must learn to assess his own capacities accurately. Each of us must consider his own financial situation. And each of us must decide what work means personally, beyond income.

15 Fun and Games

We've talked about work, which I think is very important. But there is a lot more to life: There is no reason why you can't go to movies, partake in moderate physical activities, travel, eat out, and otherwise do what other people do.

I admit, it's a violation of all expectations to be at a party and not have a glass of something in your hand. But I go anyway. At first, I went for Helen's sake, so she could have some outlet. Then, on occasion, I found something that I could eat. I feel better when I'm not totally left out. If something looks tempting, I ask Helen to taste it first. Usually she shakes her head "No." This saves me the embarrassment of not knowing what to do with whatever I've taken a bite of but can't swallow.

Dinner parties can be disastrous unless you settle the ground rules in advance. You have to explain your diet to your hosts, so you don't get served a dish smothered in mushrooms and spicy gravy, cheese-covered broccoli, and baked potatoes. Most friends will accommodate your needs. You can get away with small amounts of forbidden food on occasion, if you compensate for them until your next dialysis, or have already made room for them since your last dialysis. (Chocolate-covered bananas are off your list no matter what.) I have more trouble with fluids than with anything else at a dinner party. A little sip of water, a taste of wine, a half-cup of coffee, and I've gone beyond my day's ration, if not worse. I admonish you not to drink, but I haven't been able to follow that advice myself.

Helen and I and a group of friends have regular, rotating covered-dish dinners. Whoever prepares the main course always calls to see what I can eat. Lasagna becomes noodles and ground meat for me. Chicken pilaf becomes broiled chicken and rice. Usually, a portion of the main ingredients, before spices, gravies, mushrooms are added, suits my diet. Our friends go out of their way to make the meal attractive for me. The food may be as blah as at home; the pleasure of it comes in knowing that someone did something special.

You can eat out, but you will inevitably get more salt than you bargained for. Fast-food restaurants dispense salt and potassium as if they were the manufacturers. Chains that feature family-priced foods often presalt their meats, so you can't get salt-free main courses. At other restaurants you can get plain fish, hamburger, or steak. Tell the waiter to instruct the cook not to use spices, sauces, and dressings. The only totally worry-free foods are plain noodles and plain rice, though they're hard to find (and harder to eat).

Japanese, Chinese, and Italian restaurants are hazardous to my health. Oriental restaurants use a lot of monosodium glutamate, and Italian tomato sauce will get you for sure. Before I knew I had to limit my salt, Helen and I went to a Japanese steak house where the chef prepared the food on a grill at our table. Every time he started another portion or course, he tossed in a handful of salt. We're convinced that that meal brought my condition out into the open.

I've since discovered that renal patients can eat Japanese food if it's prepared properly. One of the doctors at our research center, whose sister-in-law is a chef on Japanese television, brought in for an office party individual portions of various tempura dishes. He brought the spices in a separate bag, so we could use them or not, as we wished. I've never tasted better food, even without the spices.

You can dine successfully at an Italian restaurant, but be careful. Even the bread may be full of garlic and salt. You may find bread sticks that are relatively salt-free, however. I've found a veal dish made with lemon-and-butter sauce; the only salt is in the butter. You can order a side dish of spaghetti with just a dab of butter and a little Parmesan cheese, which is reasonably low in salt.

I've been told that you can get Chinese food prepared without monosodium glutamate, if you ask, but I've never tried. Though I pine for their food, I've found French chefs too liberal with salt.

Probably the sneakiest salt containers are vegetables, and restaurants don't seem to be prepared to cook them separately for you. Stick to tossed salads. I've come to enjoy oil-and-vinegar dressing with a sprinkle of black pepper.

Fun isn't always food and drink, although, more often than not, these play a part. Recreation is getting away from what you normally do or see. It's a change of pace.

One day, one of my renal patients failed to show up for an appointment. Eventually, we learned that he was in the hospital. "Oh, oh," we thought, "a renal problem." No, he was riding his motorcycle and had an accident. I don't recommend that much of a change of pace, but he did get away from it all. Another patient told me he dialyzes from 1:00 to 5:00 each morning because he likes to talk on his C.B. radio until 1 A.M. His recreation is more sedentary. Quite a few patients install dialysis machines in houseboats and mobile homes. One wealthy patient, I am told, installed one machine in his yacht and one in his home. He leaves a third in the dialysis center for his use whenever he comes to town.

Helen loves to travel. Before I became ill, we had some very wonderful trips. It's harder now, but we've learned we can do it. Because my work requires travel, I was forced to overcome my anxieties and venture into the world.

The first trip I took was to a meeting in Orlando, Florida. Helen and I drove there with our two boys. Through the travel guide published by NAPHT (see Chapter 8), we had arranged to dialyze at a center in Orlando. It was a bit scary, putting my life in the hands of absolute strangers. Fortunately, it worked out well. The people were friendly and efficient, and the TV worked. At that time, I was accustomed to using an anesthetic before getting the needle. In this center, they didn't believe in it; they just inserted the fistula needles. As I mumbled, "Wait! What about Xylocaine?" the nurse popped it in with no more discomfort than I had with an anesthetic. Since then, I've never used Xylocaine again.

With that very pleasant start, I got the courage to visit other places. I found some good centers and some bad, but I've survived them all.

Some patients have told me that it's hard to get into dialysis centers in popular vacation areas. We vacationed at a South Carolina resort one year. The nearest center was in Savannah, Georgia, 90 minutes away over back roads. It started its first shift at 6:30 in the morning. We rose at 5:00 and rushed off into the darkness of early morning. The family toured Savannah while I dialyzed. It took me several hours to recover from each run, so we spent two full days of vacation on dialysis. It was so wonderful a vacation that it was worth the trouble of the trips.

We know we can travel the big cities and stay at resorts reasonably close to cities with dialysis centers, but we want to get away. Some day, I'll go portable. I'll get a suitcase kidney and cut my leash to centers completely.

Recreation often means interacting with people. Don't let your illness make others feel uncomfortable. If it does, they'll avoid you in the future. This doesn't mean that you can't let them know your special needs or limitations, but you have to realize that you may be a strange creature to them. You live with ESRD every day; they don't. What's taken for granted by others is critical for you. For example, people pop in at work to see if I want a cup of coffee. They don't realize they're tempting me. The same people might ask a reformed alcoholic if he wants a drink. One of the physicians with whom I had lunch one day was going over the menu with me as we waited for the waiter.

"The grilled cheese looks good," he said.

"Can't eat it."

"How about the spaghetti and meat sauce?"

"Can't eat it."

"Well, try the potato pancakes."

"Can't eat 'em."

"Looks as if you'll just have a glass of water. There isn't anything else you can have."

"Can't drink it."

He didn't understand, just like most people.

Often people talk about zipping off to some place for the weekend, leaving Friday night and returning Sunday night. Or they say, "Let's go to the movies tonight and to dinner tomorrow night." They don't understand that, with night-time dialysis, I can't just pick up and go, nor can I go out two nights in a row during the week without rearranging a whole week's dialysis schedule. You need to explain to people why you can't do what they'd like to do, so they'll understand and not feel you're avoiding them.

Often you've got to be the one to take the first step socially, because people may not know how to react to you. But once you've taken that step, the rest will come much more easily. It's also important to you, as well as to others, that your conversations deal with the things that interest the group. If you were to talk only about your illness and problems, you'd quickly bore everyone to tears. People can't relate for very long to your strange world. Be prepared to listen. They have problems, too. Yours may be worse, but don't play "Can you top this?"

Remember that you're a salesperson for the ESRD program. The taxpayers are spending over a billion dollars per year to keep us alive. If people see you cheerful and enjoying life, they'll know it's worth the price. If you're a grump who just sits and complains, people may wonder why they're spending so much money on our dialysis.

16 Doctors, Nurses, and Other Powerful Personnel

Once upon a time, we all believed that the President was above reproach, that all policemen were good guys, and that doctors dispensed remedies out of an infinite wisdom they shared with God. I know too much about doctors to believe they are all-knowing and infallible. That is why I'm perplexed when I see patients looking at physicians with awe.

In a way, it's understandable. Dialysis puts you in a dependent position. You lie on a couch surrounded by mysterious equipment that sucks up your blood, swishes it around, and spits it back. Meanwhile, the center's staff members flit around from couch to couch. You don't know what they are doing and they don't tell you, so you assume it is something significant. Since they know so much and you know so little, you begin to view them with awe.

When the BOSS enters the center, everyone snaps to attention. You lie there, waiting for the doctor to make his way to your couch. Then it's your turn in the limelight. For a couple minutes, you get to ask all the questions you can remember from the mental list you have made. A smile, a nod, and he moves on. No wonder he appears God-like. Besides, he's your lifeline. You look to him to keep you alive.

While it's reasonable to turn to a physician for medical advice, many people think that the doctor has it in his power to keep them perfectly healthy. There is no doctor who can keep you "in good health." He can only tell you what you have to do. That itching will stop if *you* watch what you eat and take your medications. Your weight will stay down if *you* watch your fluids. That dialysis machine does only what it's made to do. The rest is up to you, not your doctor.

You can expect certain things from your center and the doctor in charge. Naturally, you can expect them to be friendly, kind, courteous, and cheerful, but they should also be competent. I've visited several centers and have had a mix of experiences. At one place, all the patients looked ill; I never saw the doctor there. You'd think that he'd come by to say hello to a visiting physician, but there I was, the first time in his center, and he just left everything up to his staff. He sent me a bill for his services, however, and, though I was there for only two runs, he insisted on ordering lab work, for which I was also charged. My dialysis was a disaster. I gained 10 pounds that week, even though I ate almost exclusively at the home of a friend who was extraordinarily careful—probably more careful than Helen—about preparing salt-free food. I've a pretty good idea about that center.

Your physician should see you regularly—if just briefly—no less often than every two months. You ought to see him making rounds while you are dialyzing. You ought to have a chance to discuss your medical situation with him. Your problems should not stop with the nurse. Don't get me wrong. The nurse should know if you have a problem, and the nurse may solve your problem without seeing the doctor. But if you feel you need to discuss the problem with the doctor, he ought to be available within a reasonable time.

I'm fortunate. My nephrologist is interested in whatever troubles his patients. He phones employers if his patients have difficulties on the job. He contacts suppliers for his home patients. He attends NAPHT meetings. Not everyone is like that, but it'd be nice if they were.

The Federal government has established requirements that centers must meet to be eligible for Medicare. Patient groups, like NAPHT, can form their own watchdog committees to see that centers improve the quality of their operations. The committees can visit centers and get the patients' views of how things are going. The watchdog group can see if the patients are treated well, if the equipment is in good working order, whether patients' questions are answered, whether the doctor sees all the patients regularly, and things of a similar nature.

A smart doctor finds a good dialysis nurse and puts her in charge of the day-to-day operations of the dialysis program. I learned long ago that an experienced nurse can be a great source of medical and supervisory wisdom. Some of them can get their advice across quietly, so the M.D. still looks as if he's on the ball.

Under the nurse's supervision are LPNs and technicians who check blood pressure and other vital signs, troubleshoot the machines, and run much of the actual dialysis.

A dietician is likely to appear just as you're about to bite into the pickle you smuggled into the center. You may resent them at first, because they always seem to want to take something off your allowed list. After a while, you learn to hate what they do instead of them personally. You'll find that a good dietician not only spells out a diet in grams and calories, but helps you live with your diet.

Social workers go with dialysis centers as does mustard with franks. And well they should. If anyone has a spectrum of problems to deal with, it's you and your family. Social workers are listeners; they're people you should find it easiest to pour your troubles on. They can provide counseling, guide you to financial help, direct you to others who can help in other ways, and perform other useful services.

Some centers have psychologists who evaluate and help you cope with emotional problems.

A center's staff can find a great deal of stress in their work. After all, they're responsible for people's lives. No matter how long they've been on the job, they may still feel guilt if something goes wrong.

Health professionals experience ambivalence in their work. They want their patients to get well. If they don't get well, the professionals may get depressed and hostile. It's as if they were to say to a patient, "How dare you not get better when I take care of you?" On the other hand, if the patient gets too much better he won't need them. It's like parents wanting a child to grow up and be independent, yet fearing that the child *will* become independent and leave.

Some staff members develop a God-complex. *They* know what's best. They make the value judgments for you, based on their own standards: "If you'd stop hanging around with those drinking buddies of yours, you'd be better off." True, but perhaps these are lifelong friends, and their companionship is important to you. "You'll be much better off with a job." Most of the people who work in dialysis centers believe in work. It's important to them, and so they feel it's important to you. (I'm that way, and I'm always startled when I learn that someone else isn't.) They should realize that work may be threatening to you because it points out how much less you can do now that you're ill.

Staff members like to psychologize. It's one of their favorite pastimes. "John Tippler drinks too much fluid because he's rebeling against authority." "Molly Muerta doesn't take her medicine because she's suicidal." "Robert Gutterman tells dirty jokes because he's impotent and he's trying to hide it." Maybe they're right, maybe they're wrong, but once the staff puts you in such a psychological pigeon hole, it's hard to get out.

Doctors, Nurses, and Other Powerful Personnel

Among the most irritating things medical people do to patients—I do it too—is to talk down to them. "Why don't you just lie down, and we'll take care of you." The next patronizing dietician who sing-songs to me, "We're going to have to cut out eating our bananas," is going to get one of our bananas stuffed up our nose.

The staff can become attached to patients. While on a trip, I was dialyzing for a week in a center I had never been to before. Everyone was gloomy. No one said anything. It was like a funeral. Most centers are so cheerful it's almost irritating if you aren't feeling good. Near the end of the first dialysis run, I stopped one LPN. "What's the matter?" I asked. "Did someone on the staff die?" She look startled, but said nothing. Two days later, when I came back, I learned that two patients had suddenly and unexpectedly died on the weekend. The staff had been unconsciously in mourning.

Patients play their own games, sometimes to gain attention, sometimes to make trouble. One trick is to "tattle" on another patient to appear better by comparison. "Sara Cervalat was eating salami. That's terrible. I'd never cheat like that." Most centers have a patient who always calls for help: "Fix this pillow. Tilt my chair. Check this needle." A hundred small requests just to get attention. Some patients try to get different staff members to answer the same question differently. Then they play one against the other to get an "official" O.K. to do something they're afraid they shouldn't do, or to manipulate one into embarrassment.

A good center features an educational program for its patients. A good center is one that isn't afraid of what you know, only that you don't know enough. I'm appalled at the number of patients who know little or nothing about dialysis. Perhaps it's not because they aren't interested.

17

Rules for Worry

It used to be that tomorrow was automatic. You didn't wonder whether you'd see the next day; you knew you would. You didn't wonder if you'd be alive for your daughter's graduation; you just wondered if you could afford it. With ESRD, the horizon doesn't hold an automatic tomorrow. There are no guarantees.

You may have worked at your job for 20 years, and now, suddenly, it's no longer secure. You may have begun to feel comfortable financially. Now, finances are a nightmare. There's a lot more to worry about than you've ever had before. It's not surprising, then, that ESRD patients and their families are anxious, depressed, and nervous.

I worry about each dialysis. Will I get cramps? Will it remove enough fluid so I can drink my miserable 16 ounces per day? I worry about each needle stick; I worry about my monthly lab reports. Besides ESRD worries, I'm also subject to the whole range of normal concerns. I don't retreat into a corner, though, and suck my thumb—it's not salt-free.

I've managed to handle my burdens to some degree; otherwise, I'd be committed to an institution. With all the "how to do it" books around, there probably is one about how to worry, but I've developed my own approaches to handling things that bother me.

When we become ill, we pay more attention to our bodies and their functions. Before ESRD, how much water did you drink? Most of us couldn't answer that question precisely. Now, drinking water is a major event to be carefully planned and executed. You sip it to savor it, let it linger on your tongue, and calculate every drop.

Every time you visit the doctor, you are questioned about your body and its functions. How have your bowel movements been? How much urine do you pass? Even the weigh-in before and after dialysis reinforces your concern with yourself. Each meal serves to remind you that you have to watch your intake.

It is not surprising that you soon become centered on yourself. You *have* to in order to survive, but the more attention you pay to yourself, the more you worry about every little variation from your daily routine.

You can't stop paying attention to yourself, but you can keep perspective. I realize that I'm variable. I'm not going to be the same each day, so I don't get upset about it. We can tolerate minor variations, but major changes require attention. A temperature of 98.7° F. wouldn't alarm us, but 102° F. should. Today I have no appetite. Am I uremic? If I don't have an appetite for a week, then I worry.

My second rule is that worry doesn't accomplish anything. Action does. You can worry for years about getting fat, but unless you cut down on calories you'll get fatter. You can worry that you will die, but that won't stop you from dying. You can worry whether some food has too much salt, but that won't lower its salt content.

Do something about what worries you. If you're worried

about death, do everything you can to reduce the risks of death. Watch your diet, take your medicine, listen to your medical advisor, and look both ways when you cross the street. If you're worried about the salt content of a piece of food, don't eat it. Then you won't have to worry about it. When you've done everything you can to eliminate the cause of your worries, then what happens is out of your hands. So why worry any longer about it?

Getting out of yourself is the next maneuver on my "down with worry" list. If you center on yourself when you are sick, then part of getting well is shifting your attention away from yourself. The more you become active and involved with people, groups, things, the less you are wrapped up in yourself. When does a toothache bother you most? If you're doing something that takes most of your attention, you may even forget all about it, but when you're not distracted, the pain grows. In the same way, when you're involved in activities unrelated to your illness, you're less concerned with it.

In general, despite your problems, you must stay active. When you're physically inactive, your muscles weaken and your joints get stiff. If you lie down most of the time, you'll get dizzy when you try to stand. If you're intellectually inactive and think only about yourself, you'll exaggerate your own problems. If you fail to be socially active, no one'll visit or invite you out anymore. You become isolated.

When I ache all over and concentrate on my patients, my miseries fade. When I worry about them, I'm not worrying about me. I'd much rather worry about someone else's problems; I can send them away if they get to be too much.

When all these tricks fail, and I still worry, I have one left: I think about other people and ask myself, "Would I really trade places with. . . .?" Most of the time, the other guy has problems I wouldn't want.

It comes down to whether you like yourself. If you do, then you can tolerate the things that make you what you are.

On Borrowed Time: Living With Hemodialysis

You can even look positively at the things that cause you pain and worry. Dialysis is no fun, but it's also a fantastic experience shared by very few human beings. And you're fortunate enough to develop ESRD when dialysis is available. A few years ago—and even now in some countries—you'd have died. You've conquered death, if only temporarily. That's amazing. You've had the strength and the courage to meet a life-threatening crisis and come out on top. Pat yourself on the back, you've earned it. And don't forget: Things are changing so rapidly that better times are just around the corner.

Before I became ill, I worked with the handicapped. I always told my patients not to give up, but I wondered what I'd do in their place. Would I have the guts to pick myself up and overcome a handicap? Now I know.

18 Just for Diabetics

You've had diabetes for years, and now, on top of that, you've got ESRD. Join the group. It's estimated that one fourth to one third of all ESRD patients are diabetics. You definitely are not alone. But you are fortunate. A few years ago, diabetics were rejected for hemodialysis and transplantation. Even now in England, the national health system will not accept diabetics for hemodialysis.

When I first learned I had to go on dialysis, my nephrologist scared me halfway back to health by describing all the horrible things that might happen to the diabetic on hemodialysis. Now he doesn't hesitate to recommend dialysis to a diabetic; he's had some very good experiences.

Times change and medicine progresses. In fact, by the time you read this, the chapter on the future may be the past! I'll try to tell it "like it is" for now. As you already know, it can be pretty rough.

Diabetics get into renal problems in various ways. They

are subject to infections, and this includes kidney infection. Diabetes can affect both large and small blood vessels in many organs, including the kidney. And diabetes can attack kidney tissue directly.

If you've been dependent on insulin since childhood—a juvenile diabetic—the odds are 50:50 that you'll have ESRD after 20 years of diabetes. For people who get diabetes later in life, ESRD is less likely. When your doctor first detects evidence that you have renal disease, he already knows that in five years you'll be at the end-stage. It's inevitable. It's estimated that from 2,500 to 3,000 diabetics die of kidney disease each year.

Diabetics develop other problems in addition to kidney failure. They're likely to have eye problems; diabetes is one of this country's leading causes of blindness. Body imbalances created by failing kidneys add to the loss of vision. Moreover, the high blood pressure that kidney disease and diabetes bring on can also cause eye damage. Even after beginning dialysis, a number of diabetics continue to lose vision. Some, however, improve. There is some reason to hope that transplantation may stabilize vision, though it's not likely to improve it.

Often, nerve and muscle damage accompany blindness. Both diabetes and the poisons that accumulate because of kidney disease can damage the nerves. Sometimes it's hard to tell which disease is causing the nerve injury. When dialysis has had a chance to clean up the body, some damage to the nerve that the kidney disease caused may be reversed. However, the damage due to diabetes may get worse.

I can recall the slow breakdown of my nerve function. At first, I felt a slight numbness in my soles and toes. It didn't hurt to grasp my foot and squeeze it hard, but a light moving sensation felt very strange. I couldn't stand sheets or blankets on my feet or the eerie sensation that came when I pulled on my socks. Still, I had no weakness and could walk forever. I used to ride an exercycle five or more miles each evening. How far I had lost feeling became apparent after I broke the nail on my great toe while riding the exercycle. The first time I broke half the toenail, and I didn't discover it until I got ready for bed. A few days later, I broke the other half. Each time, I didn't feel anything.

As time went on, I was unaware of much change until one day I tried to climb the stands at my son's junior league football field. After one or two large steps, one thigh felt all cramped up. One weekend, after shopping at a mall for about an hour, I started back to my car. Both legs refused to move; they were like boards. Somehow, I made it to my car, but I had to rest for 15 to 20 minutes before I could control my legs well enough to drive.

As my combined diseases progressed, my muscles were wasting away. The edema fluid from my kidney failure puffed up my skin and concealed the wasting. While in San Francisco for a meeting, Helen and I went sightseeing one day. A friendly passerby said it was just a nice walk to a tower from which we could get a good view of the city. What he didn't say was that it was almost straight up. By the thirteenth set of stairs, I thought I'd die: My legs were knotted terribly. Despite these warnings, I didn't think I was becoming paralyzed—just overworking my muscles. But when I collapsed just getting out of bed, I couldn't deny it any longer. I finally went to see a physician.

Ironically, at my medical center, there were two or three doctors who ran special tests on nerves and muscles. I was one of them. Many patients have suffered through these tests at my hands, and now it was my turn. The tests were uncomfortable, I knew, but what worried me most was whether I'd be able to "take it" the way I gave it out.

Actually, I slept through almost the whole thing. I was so ill by then that I kept dozing off. I couldn't feel the pin pricks and electric impulses. My honor was saved. Now I tell my patients, "I've had these same tests. They didn't bother me a bit. I even slept through them. So just relax."

Other nerves become affected. The nerves that supply muscles in the trunk (back and stomach wall), the hips and thighs, and the shoulders may be damaged temporarily. This type of damage (called amyotrophy) tends to clear up with good diabetic control.

The nerves supplying your blood vessels, stomach, intestines, and bladder may also not function correctly. You may suffer nausea and vomiting, and, alternately, diarrhea and constipation. Kidney disease can also cause these problems, so you often don't know which is doing it. You *do* know to whom, however!

The bladder normally stretches like a balloon. But with nerve damage, the bladder loses its elasticity: It doesn't resist the stretching. You may have difficulty passing water until your bladder fills up considerably. That happened to me at a time when my kidney was pouring out large amounts of urine. The problem came to a very unpleasant conclusion. My muscle weakness concerned my doctor, so he decided to have the surgeon take a small piece of muscle (a muscle biopsy), so he could study it under the microscope. To ease the pain, my doctor gave me some medication, which eased my pain all right, but also completely paralyzed my bladder. I couldn't urinate. Finally, I was catheterized (a small tube was inserted into the bladder). More than three pints drained off. It was days before I knew whether I'd need a permanent catheter. I'd never been so distressed.

When nerve control of the blood vessels isn't working right, the vessels don't contract and relax properly. Usually when you stand up, the blood vessels in your legs contract and build up resistance so that your blood doesn't drain into your legs. If blood pools in your legs, your blood pressure drops, and your brain doesn't get enough blood. You get dizzy or lightheaded and may faint. It's particularly difficult when you get up quickly. The room may spin, and you can feel the blood drain from your face. A peculiar hollow feeling sickens your stomach, and you feel clammy. It may be difficult to distinguish the reaction from insulin shock. Often you feel better when you eat something, which leads you to think it was an insulin reaction. However, you sit down to eat, and it could be the sitting down that made you feel better, not the food, so you're still not sure.

Anemia accounts for a good part of the fatigue you feel. You're used to feeling tired when your blood sugar goes out of whack, but this new fatigue is beyond anything you've felt before. You can't even test your urine for sugar and get an accurate result. So it's more difficult to know whether your symptoms of headache, fatigue, shakiness, dizziness, or lightheadedness are due to your variations in blood sugar, a falling blood pressure, or too much fluid loss on dialysis.

Diabetics with kidney disease are also more likely to have heart disease and strokes, inflammation of the lining of the heart (pericarditis), and assorted infections. While approximately one half of all patients on dialysis for more than five years die of heart and blood vessel disease, more than 60 per cent of all diabetics on dialysis die of these causes.

Overall, diabetics have done well on dialysis. The ordinary dialysis patient has about a 70 per cent chance of being alive three years after beginning dialysis; the diabetic has perhaps a 25 per cent chance. With increasing success of transplantation, there is a trend toward advising diabetics to obtain transplants.

Since I've been on dialysis, kidney transplants for diabetics with renal disease have gone from experimental or "I'm not sure it's the best thing" approach to a "it's looking better and better." The best statistics on survival of the patient and the donated kidney come from the Midwest. Other centers haven't achieved a high success rate yet. Some specialists are so encouraged about transplants, that, instead of having the patient go on dialysis first and then get a new kidney, they suggest getting a transplant before the patient needs dialysis.

Even so, chances of success with diabetics are less than

with other ESRD patients, and the donated kidney will not function as well in a diabetic as it would in a nondiabetic. Diabetics have more complications and a rougher follow-up period, too. And diabetes may damage the transplanted kidney as it did the original kidney. A return to a fuller, more normal life is much more likely with a transplant than with dialysis, however. You and your physician have to assess the pluses and minuses for you personally.

These are the grim facts. Yet, here I am, partially paralyzed in my hands and feet, having been paralyzed in my trunk, hips, and shoulders as well, on dialysis and thriving. I teach medicine, see patients, do research, and write both scientific and nonscientific materials. My wife still tolerates me, my children—at least one—still listen to me, and we even manage to travel and have fun. It's obvious that you can survive. The question is how. One person's solution may not be another's, but there are some basic principles that apply to almost everyone.

No matter how loose you may have been on your diabetic diet, you've got to stick to your new dietary restrictions. It's not easy. You've no way to test yourself by urine as you may have done before. As noted, you often can't tell whether a headache is from low blood sugar, low blood pressure, or dialysis. Before, you could guzzle diet drinks, munch as much celery, carrots, and other low-calorie goodies as you wished. Now you've got to watch carbohydrates, sodium, potassium, phosphates, as well as fluids. When your blood sugar goes up, you get thirsty, but if you drink, you retain too much fluid. Your body's ability to use fats also gets messed up, and this leads to heart and blood vessel problems.

To complicate things further, your insulin requirements may change when your kidneys fail and when you begin dialysis. You and your physician will have to monitor your condition carefully. Your blood sugar levels may not give. you the same clues that they used to.

Low blood sugar used to make me irritable and shaky,

with a peculiar pounding in the pit of my stomach. Sometimes it was accompanied by a headache. Since going on dialysis, I still get these reactions, but, at times, low blood sugar produces nausea instead. High blood sugar levels used to make me thirsty, make me urinate a great deal, and make me tired. Now I'm always thirsty, rarely urinate, and am often tired anyway. The other day my blood sugar rose to 700, and I was only tired. The next morning, I woke up at 5:00 in insulin shock. I've never been that brittle before.

With diabetes, you always were subject to foot problems. Now, when your nerves aren't working so well and swelling may make it easier for your feet to be injured, it's especially important to pay attention to nail care, athlete's foot, and pressure areas. Calluses act as pressure points and reduce the blood supply to tissues under the callus.

At the time of this writing, I have a cumbersome cast on one leg from my knee to my toes. It takes the pressure off my toes, so that an ulcer on one toe can heal. The whole problem started simply. For some reason—a wrinkle in my sock or something equally minor—I developed a blister on my toe. The area got infected. The toe swelled, putting more pressure on the tissues. The infection wouldn't heal.

We used a potent antibiotic given by vein while I was on dialysis. The infection responded, but the ulcer wouldn't close. For eight or nine months, it'd heal and then break open again. Finally, after the area became reinfected, we tried the cast. With repeated infections like this, there's a danger that I'll lose my leg. One toe has done more to slow me down and limit my activities than ESRD and diabetes.

It's important that you get into the habit of checking your feet each night to look for redness, blisters, cracks in the skin, and calluses. In general, since you are subject to all sorts of medical problems (eyes, nerves, blood vessels), and since these problems may progress faster when you're on dialysis, you must be particularly careful to keep a regular pattern of check-ups with your doctor.

19 The Cost of It All

Once a year, I count up what it costs me—above what Medicare pays—to be on dialysis, so I can complete my medical tax deductions. The total amounts are staggering. For the average in-center dialysis patient it costs $25,000 to $30,000 for a year's hemodialysis. A home patient runs one third to one half the cost. Estimates of national costs run to $1 billion for about 40,000 dialysis and transplant patients in 1977—there'll be more in the future.

It's frightening. It's frightening because I don't know how long this nation will be willing to support such an expensive program. Frightening because the cost given is just the tip of the iceberg. What about the tax income lost from nonworking patients? What about Social Security payments for disability? What about the profiteering in supplies, equipment, and fees? It is easy to file a claim with Medicare, Medicaid, and all the rest, but it eventually comes out of someone's pocket. Uncle Sam's pocket is us.

On Borrowed Time: Living With Hemodialysis

Is it possible to decide that someone's life costs too much? Should you have to demonstrate that you are worthy to be kept alive? In the beginning, when hemodialysis was available for only a few, committees decided who could go on hemodialysis and who would not. The patient had to carry the full cost of hemodialysis or transplantation. To be eligible for financial aid, patients had to first use up their savings and sell their property. Then, in 1973, Medicare coverage was extended to ESRD patients under 65 years of age through the End-Stage Renal Disease Program. The impact on the care of ESRD patients has been dramatic.

With money available to pay for treatments, more artificial kidney machines became available, more dialysis units were established, and more physicians became interested in ESRD. Research flourished, and technology advanced rapidly, mainly because of money. People who would have been denied dialysis were accepted because machines and personnel were available and payment was guaranteed.

Is this outpouring of national monies cost-effective? We don't know. Home dialysis is probably more cost-effective than in-center dialysis, and a successful transplant is more cost-effective (about $20,000 for a transplant plus $5,000 a year for continued care) than either of the two dialysis sites. We don't know yet what the total cost picture really is. Certainly, inflation drives dialysis costs up just as it drives up costs in every other aspect of our lives.

There were some situations built into the 1973 legislation that defeated cost effectiveness. While home dialysis is less expensive than in-center dialysis, there has been a financial advantage to dialyze in-center. First, the nonpatient would-be dialysis partner can more readily hold a job. With your spouse at work, you don't lose disability benefits, even though there is a regular income for the family. Since Medicare—and in some cases, Medicaid also—covers your costs, why should you care how much a center charges? It isn't coming out of your pocket. Center costs are so high, that the

112

20 per cent that Medicare doesn't cover is often waived. In fact, until current legislation, Medicare didn't cover the cost of some supplies for home dialysis. Home patients wound up paying as much as 40 per cent of the total cost of dialysis. So, while home dialysis is less expensive overall, it cost the patient more. Moreover, physicians earn more from in-center patients than they do from patients who dialyze at home. I have to believe that some physicians may encourage in-center dialysis because it's more profitable for them.

In addition, to dialyze at home, you need to buy or rent equipment—a dialysis lounge, for example—and you need plumbing work done. Also, your utility bills are higher. To train for home dialysis, you spend about one month learning theory and techniques. If you trained before the first day of your third month of dialysis, you weren't yet covered under Medicare. Helen and I trained before I was covered, and it cost me more than $2,000.

It's no surprise that the percentage of ESRD patients who dialyze at home dropped from 40 per cent in 1970 to less than 10 per cent. The most recent ESRD legislation, however, may remove some disincentives for home dialysis. The law provides a waiver of the three-month waiting period for Medicare coverage if an individual participates in a self-care training program prior to the end of the third month after the month he begins regular dialysis. ESRD patients may take advantage of the following provisions through participating dialysis centers:

● Coverage for supplies required for home dialysis.

● Coverage for services of a dialysis technician that an individual who dialyzes at home may need from time to time. These services include monitoring the patient's adaptation to self-dialysis, emergency visits where necessary, and help in installation and maintenance of equipment.

● Reimbursement of costs that a facility may incur for helping to maintain a self-dialysis unit, in which a patient can manage his own treatment with less medical supervision and assistance than is required in a full-care maintenance program.

• Reimbursement to approved dialysis facilities for the cost of dialysis equipment that is reserved for the exclusive use of entitled renal disease patients who dialyze at home. (At present, Medicare will not pay more than $50 for a piece of equipment that is purchased outright, so home patients rent equipment at much greater long-term cost.)

There may be some regulations that interpret these provisions more specifically. For a full explanation of your Medicare benefits, write to U.S. Department of H.E.W., Social Security Administration. There is a DHEW publication entitled Medicare Coverage of Kidney Dialysis and Kidney Transplant Services that you may find helpful.

Transplantation isn't cheap either. Currently, it costs about $20,000, plus $5,000 or so per year for maintenance care. Under current legislation, the patient is covered from the first day of the month he is hospitalized for transplantation, provided the transplantation surgery takes place within the next two months.)

Medicare coverage used to cease at the end of the twelfth month following transplantation. But patients may reject their kidneys even after a full year. Some don't stabilize in 12 months' time. Often, there are heavy costs in the first three years after transplantation. Medicare coverage now extends through those 36 months.

Apart from Medicare, you may be eligible for Social Security disability benefits. Find out from the social worker at any center whether you are.

Medicaid should be clearly distinguished from Medicare. Medicare is a Federal program that is uniform throughout the country. Medicaid is a Federal- and state-supported system that differs from state to state. It's designed for the poor; you are eligible only if your income is below a certain limit. Check with your social worker or your state agency to determine if you are eligible. Some states have special provisions for people whose medical bills exceed a certain proportion of their income. Check on that, also.

Many states have other financial programs for ESRD patients. Check with your social worker or your state's board of health to see if your state has such a program.

The Veterans Administration has a wide-ranging ESRD program. Eligible veterans may have better benefits than do patients on Medicare. If you're eligible for both, check them carefully to see which is better for you.

Each state has a program of rehabilitation services for disabled people, which includes ESRD patients. Your state's vocational rehabilitation program can evaluate your capabilities, test your aptitudes and interests, and provide funds for job training (including college), transportation, and even equipment and tools if needed. These programs offer job placement services. Often, homemaking is considered a vocational objective, and training for it can be covered. Ask your social worker about your state's program.

County and city governments may have programs that indirectly help ESRD patients. Some offer children and adult health services, mental health clinics, counseling programs, homemaker services, food stamps, therapy, transportation, and other adjuncts to your basic Medicare benefits. Again, your social worker is the best source of information about what's available.

The American Kidney Fund offers educational programs and may extend direct aid to patients. You may obtain information from American Kidney Fund, 7315 Wisconsin Avenue, Bethesda, Md. 20014.

Homemaker services, meals-on-wheels, and the Visiting Nurse Association all offer programs for which you may be eligible. Check with your social worker, since these programs vary from place to place.

The National Kidney Foundation (2 Park Avenue, New York, N.Y. 10016) represents the interests of renal disease patients. It helps fight the legislative battles and the national educational wars. It also supports research efforts and some local medical care programs.

Another source of information, help, comfort, and companionship is your local chapter of the National Association of Patients on Hemodialysis and Transplantation (NAPHT). The national office is at 505 Northern Boulevard, Great Neck, N.Y. 11021. It publishes NAPHT News, a patient-oriented magazine that I find interesting and helpful.

Back to taxes. I am not an accountant (if you have one, check with him), so don't rely solely on what I write here. Get the IRS booklet on medical deductions. Refer to it several times a year—not only at tax time—so you won't miss important deductions. Obviously, you deduct the actual costs to you of dialysis and other medical services, tests, and the like. Remember, you have to subtract your insurance reimbursements from your total medical costs. Don't forget to deduct insurance payments, including Medicare (Part B). You spend a fortune on drugs, so it pays to keep track of this expense. Your whole family's costs count toward your deduction. Mileage to and from doctors, dentists, centers, hospitals, can be deducted. If you travel and dialyze while away from home, travel to and from the dialysis center is deductible. Should you require an attendant to travel away from home, that person's expenses can be deducted.

The home patient can deduct for the space he uses for dialysis and for storage of supplies. This deduction includes depreciation on his home. Modifications to the room to permit dialysis and the permanent equipment purchased for dialysis are deductible.

It's a wonder why catastrophic injuries such as spinal cord injury, brain injury or stroke, coronary artery surgery and diseases such as cancer, leukemia, and hemophilia aren't covered equally with ESRD under Medicare. These disorders are also financially crippling. ESRD is a financial jungle. You can survive if you learn the safe places to rest and lick your wounds. Otherwise, the tigers will get you!

20

It Even Happens in Children

From the time I was a medical student to the present, I've never been able to steel myself against the sight of an infant in distress. It's small wonder, then, that I get disturbed when I think about infants and children with ESRD, and they make up about 10 per cent of chronic renal patients. ESRD has different effects upon them than it has on adults.

The child is in a developmental state; the structures and functions of his body and mind are changing and maturing. In general, the younger the child, the more rapidly the changes occur. "As the twig is bent, so grows the tree," the saying goes, and ESRD bends the child.

ESRD not only alters the functions and structures of the body. It also disturbs the psychological and social growth and development of the child. Because of this, the disease is more devastating to the child than to the adult. I often see people my age and say to myself, "If I were normal, I could be doing that." How terrible it must be for a child to have to have such regrets. He's never had a chance to do much of what I've already done, besides the things I'll never get to do.

Many of the technical problems of the treatment of children and infants with ESRD have to do with their size. Equipment must be small enough. Dialyzers for adults would take too much blood out of infants. They need very small dialyzers. The fluid dialyzed from an infant can't be anywhere near the amount an adult has to lose, so there have to be measurement systems that can detect small weight loss during dialysis. The infant's blood vessels are tiny, so surgeons must use special techniques to implant shunts, and only very small needles can enter the blood vessels. This is one reason many prefer peritoneal dialysis for infants.

Imagine the dietary problems with infants. Their principal food should be milk, yet milk is fluid and high in potassium, sodium, phosphates, and protein. They have to take special formulas instead of milk. And the poor guys need those awful phosphate-binding gels (like aluminum hydroxide) just as we do.

Size becomes less critical as the child gets larger, but other problems arise. Maintaining adequate nourishment is a constant problem. As you already know, the food isn't tasty. It's different from the food that other children of their age eat. My children see commercial after commercial for hamburger drive-ins, pizzas with everything, soft drinks of all kinds, candy bars, and other renal disasters. At every opportunity, they run for a snack or drink. If it's hard for an adult to restrain himself, it must be torture for a child. Like adults, many young ESRD patients don't have much appetite for foods that are allowed. Getting enough calories in safe foods into the child can be difficult.

Children with ESRD don't grow normally. They don't grow as rapidly as normal children. No one knows for certain why this happens. It may be due partly to an inadequate intake of calories, but even when enough calories are consumed, the growth rate doesn't catch up to normal.

ESRD children have slow sexual development. Puberty comes later than it does for normal children. Girls, for example, develop breasts late and menstruate late.

Bone disease is much more common in children than in adults with ESRD. Bone composition involves a complex balance of hormones, vitamin D, calcium, phosphorus, and other substances. Since children are growing, the disturbances in the bone composition are more severe than with adults. Improper bone formation may keep children from physical activity.

Like adults, children may be anemic. The anemia makes them fatigued or without endurance. This, in turn, limits their play activities, which are not only a normal part of childhood, but are how children learn about the world. Adults may take drugs to increase their blood count. These same medicines may cause children's bones to stop growing.

Children on hemodialysis are more subject to seizures or convulsions than are adults. These can frighten both children and parents. Seizures are more common when an especially large amount of fluid has to be removed at dialysis.

Children can dialyze at home, too. It's less frightening in familiar surroundings than in a center or hospital. Home dialysis can be more readily scheduled to fit in with school and other activities.

Most ESRD programs in this country orient their treatment of children toward kidney transplantation. They use dialysis as an intermediate step. Soon after beginning dialysis, preparations are made for transplantation: operations to control calcium-phosphorus balance; removal of diseased kidneys, if necessary; testing to find appropriate donors.

Transplants in children survive about as well as they do in adults. Children younger than five do less well than older children. If the new kidney functions, the child does very well. The blood count rises, bone composition improves, sexual maturation proceeds more normally, and the child feels better. Remember, however, that the child's body can reject the new kidney. Approximately one half are rejected after five years, and that's a conservative figure.

Although their condition improves after a transplant, many, if not most, children don't resume normal bone growth. This is especially true for children older than 12.

Some people think the steroids that are given after transplantation retard development. Over a long period of time they can injure and even destroy areas of bone, such as the hip. Not only can this be painful, but the patient may need surgery to remove the damaged bone.

Steroids are responsible for many other problems, also. People who take them for a long time get rounded faces, facial hair, and acne. They also develop a peculiar kind of obesity. When children develop these changes, it can be very upsetting to them and to their parents.

The psychological and social problems that ESRD children and their families have to face are perhaps the most trying part of having the disease. Adults have developed personalities, identities, have finished their educations, and have some idea of what the world is like. Children have yet to experience all these things.

The infant spends his early days developing relationships with parents and a limited number of others. It's important for him to establish a strong sense of love, security, and trust with his mother, in particular. Being held closely, sucking, and defining his body are all activities he requires so he can successfully move to the next stages of development. Dialysis, separation from his mother, the strange environment, and the other extraordinary experiences he has because of his disease all act to bend the twig.

When the child begins crawling and, later on, toddling, he is exploring his environment, learning what to touch, what things feel like, and what his abilities are. Movement is very important to the child, and he tends to get into everything. The restraints of chronic illness and dialysis are very hard on a child this age. By limiting his explorations, we limit his growth in defining who he is and what he can do. The toddler seeks independence, but dialysis forces dependence. Moreover, his parents fear injury or disease, which may complicate his already massive problems. Often, dialysis even disrupts toilet training; accidents are common during dialysis, and they embarrass the child.

You know how upset children four or five years old get whenever they scrape themselves. Seems they come running for bandages. Even little injuries upset them. Getting a shot distresses them greatly. Imagine how repeated needle sticks and the sight of all that blood can disturb a youngster.

Young children haven't a developed sense of time. Twenty minutes, 20 days, and 20 months get mixed up. You may promise that dialysis will be over in one hour, but the child may not understand an hour the same way an adult does. Often, he can't grasp that his misery will end soon. Times away from mother may seem interminable.

When the child starts school, schoolmates and friends take on great importance. Children begin to compare themselves with others. They want to do what their friends do and to be like them. Since they are smaller, weaker, chronically ill, and eat different foods, they are obviously different. Dialysis, repeated illnesses, and hospitalization interfere with classroom schedules. If they have young friends where they dialyze, this problem may not be so severe.

School children are able to understand some of the things they must endure, but often they're not told what they should know in language they can understand. Children are curious; their intellects are eagerly growing. If the dialysis staff don't respond properly, they can stifle this curiosity.

Teenagers are difficult even when they're normal. They're self-conscious, unsure of their masculinity and femininity, and they undergo radical body changes. ESRD delays their growth, delays sexual maturation, and causes other obvious differences (such as pallor) between them and their classmates, all of which can upset their already fragile self-esteem. Social life is very important, and, unfortunately, revolves around junk food to a large degree. Diet restrictions and the time dialysis takes disrupt the social process.

Teenagers are constitutionally rebellious. For them, authority is to be ignored or destroyed. But they can't successfully rebel against the restrictions that ESRD imposes. If a teenager isn't difficult to work with, he's likely to be dependent and passive—a good patient, but not much else.

Most families have troubles that simmer like a pot of water on a stove. Along comes ESRD, and it's like turning up the burner. Now the water boils. Money gradually becomes scarce. Luxuries like vacations, a new car, a new piece of furniture, or eating out are no longer affordable. Parents may begin to bicker over the budget.

Time, like money, is a limited commodity. If you spend six hours with one child, you can't spend that time with another child, your spouse, or on things that need doing. Siblings become envious, and the husband may resent his wife's exclusive preoccupation with the sick child.

The family may become isolated. While the parents spend more time with the sick child and less time out where they'd spend money, they socialize less. Siblings may stop bringing friends home.

Parents become "too tired," and cut down sexual activity, cease displaying affection, limit family activities. Weak marriages may fall apart.

Even with transplantation, the families must live with the fear of rejection of the new kidney. The complications are a source of concern. With reduced ability to fight infections, every minor childhood illness is cause for alarm.

Under the weight of all these stresses, some ESRD children become behavioral problems. They may resist treatment, become hostile, destructive, or find some other way to vent their anger and frustration. This behavior can further strain the family structure.

Despite all the interruptions in a normal school schedule, it's important that the educational process continue, not only providing information, but also permitting social growth, developing self-esteem, and preparing the child for a choice of a career. The teacher often has to be a counselor as well. Be wary of teachers who recommend home tutoring. It may be that the teacher can't cope with the problems of a chronically ill child. In general, the benefits of belonging to the school community outweigh the advantage of fewer problems with home tutoring.

As the child grows, career choices become more important. The child may have been living from dialysis to dialysis, but now he must expand his horizons. ESRD or not, the child becomes an adult, and must live in an adult world.

21 We All Must Die

I know I'll die. That doesn't worry me anymore, not since I've been on borrowed time. What I am concerned about, though, is how and when I'll die. Like most people, I don't like painful, drawn out, and miserable deaths, or messy ones. I'd much prefer a bolt-of-lightning-type affair—wham, bam, and it's over! It's rough on those who are left, but it seems an easier way to go.

Most of all, I'm concerned with when. There are people I need to protect, and I've determined to do everything I can for them before my time comes. That's why there's so much to do before I go.

One of the first things I did when I learned I was in chronic renal failure was to see my lawyer and estate planner. I was too late, really: Due to the obvious nature of my disease, I'd already lost some options. If you can, be prepared for any medical catastrophe. Get your insurance and estate plans lined up. Most of us wait, of course, and then bemoan our procrastination. Even if you've just been diagnosed, you can still do some planning.

A growing number of people are writing living wills, documents in which you can indicate that you don't want to prolong your life beyond the point at which survival would be a semihuman condition. You'd probably want to discuss a document like this, in advance, with your physician, rabbi or minister, lawyer, and family. In some states, it's considered a legal document. A friend has permitted me to reproduce her living will as an example.

To My Family, My Physicians, My Church, and the Executors of My Will:

If the time comes when I can no longer take part in decisions for my own future, let this statement stand as the testament of my wishes.

If there is no reasonable expectation of my recovery from physical or mental disability, I, _____, request that I be allowed to die and not be kept alive by artificial means or heroic measures. I believe that insofar as is possible, I have the same right of control over my death as I have had over my life. I do not fear death, but I do fear irreversible deterioration and hopeless pain. I ask that medication be mercifully administered for terminal suffering even if it hastens the moment of death. This request is based on two firm convictions: one, the inestimable value of life so long as it is useful in fulfillment of God's purpose; and second, a belief in God's gift of life after death.

I make this statement after careful consideration and with the full knowledge of all to whom it is addressed. Although this document is not legally binding, I hope you will feel morally bound to follow its wishes. I recognize that this request places a heavy burden upon you, and I write it with the intention of sharing that responsibility with you.

_____

Signature

_____

Signature of nearest relative

_____

Signature of clergyman

_____

Date

People don't like to talk about death. Doctors find it difficult to tell a patient he's going to die. Family members get upset when they have to talk about death to someone in the family when he's dying. With everyone so somber and hushed when someone is near death, children may come to regard it as strange and mysterious.

We instinctively avoid death. It's as if we feel we're immortal even when we know we must die. You're sad when someone dies, but deep down you're grateful that it wasn't you. Survivors often feel guilt. "Why didn't I do more?" "If only I had known how to spot his trouble earlier." There's always something we've left undone, always some effort we could have made, but didn't.

We even avoid the word. "He has passed away." "He's gone to heaven." "God has taken him." We cushion death's impact with floral wreaths, ceremonies, and monuments. We dress and decorate our corpses, encase them in extravagant boxes that will keep them "forever," and carefully, splendidly place them in the ground. For whom? Not for the one who has died, but for the living. To soothe our guilt, ease our own fear of death, and provide an opportunity for public grieving. The rituals are cathartic. They may be very useful, but they're for the living, not the dead.

ESRD patients are kept alive by machines. We should have died, yet we live, if only temporarily. It's strange to feel so alive, yet to know I should be dead.

Over the past few years, a small number of physicians and psychologists have begun to study the emotional reactions of the dying patient. They have identified stages through which the dying pass. Since many of us have gone through some of these stages before dialysis or transplantation intervened, you may recognize some of the reactions.

Shock characterizes the first stage. When you learn of your fate you become confused. Your sense of immortality is crushed. No longer can you think of death as happening to the other guy; it's going to happen to you. The reaction is similar to the one that comes on learning you have ESRD. The dying move quite naturally from this stage into the stage of denial and isolation.

Disbelief in the doctor's prognosis is one form of denial. "No, not me. It can't be. I'm too young. These tests are wrong. You've confused me with another patient. There's an error in the lab reports." Patients may go doctor shopping to see if a different doctor will give them another answer. The patient often becomes isolated. Family and friends who know the patient's reaction don't talk to him about it. The patient evades the issue. People begin to avoid the patient so that the subject won't come up. Soon the patient becomes isolated and may develop an intense sense of loneliness.

Eventually, denial changes into anger. Instead of saying, "No, it can't be," he begins to ask, "Why me?" Often he directs his anger toward others. "Those lousy doctors don't do anything for me." "You can call those nurses, but no one comes." "My wife doesn't really care, or she would've visited me sooner." Anger may take the form of envy at the good fortune of others. "He's lucky. He's got a good job, money, and a family. I've never had it as good as he does."

As anger fades, the patient begins to bargain for just a little more time. "Doc, just keep me going 'til after my kid graduates." "I'll stick to my diet and take my medication if you just get me to that wedding. I'll do anything you say." Often, the bargaining is with God. "Let me live and I'll be the best person you ever saw." "Give me another chance, God, and I'll do what's right."

When bargaining fails and the certainty of his fate is evident, the patient becomes depressed. He grieves not only over what he's lost, but also over what won't be. He may have been a physically active person, and he grieves for his lost strength and agility. But he also may grieve that his children must grow up without a father or that his wife must live without a husband. He may regret the goals that are now out of his reach. "If this hadn't happened, I could've moved up in this company." "I was going to buy a place in the country, but now . . ."

Slowly, the patient comes to accept death. He knows he'll die, he's exhausted all appeals. He loses the strong feelings about death he had before. He's less interested in things other than his death and its effects on others. At this point he may seek seclusion to quietly prepare for death.

Through all these stages, hope lingers in the background. No matter how slim, there's always the chance his sentence will be reprieved: There will be a breakthrough in medical science and he'll be saved. I don't know if hope ever completely dies.

These stages are not all that different from those we go through on our way way to accepting the fact of ESRD (see Chapter 2). In ESRD, a part of us has died. We've grieved for the loss and have come to accept a new form of life. Fortunately, we now can reasonably expect to live, not die. However, one day, perhaps soon, we will die.

On Borrowed Time: Living With Hemodialysis

What happens to the family while the patient struggles with death and dying? Certainly, it goes through some process of its own. Let's assume that the family genuinely loves the person who's dying; otherwise, there are too many possible reactions. They're sorry to see him die, but they don't want him to suffer. They want him to live, but they also want him to be at peace. Because they feel that death would be good, the family members feel guilty.

They feel guilty, too, when they enjoy themselves while someone they love is dying. At the same time, they may resent the problems the dying person causes. They can't plan anything that'd disrupt normal routine in a major way, such as a trip, because the person may die at any time. Children may resent a dying parent abandoning them. A wife may resent a dying husband leaving her with all the responsibility to care for the house and family. Even before death comes, the family will worry about their future needs. How will we live? Will there be enough money?

Death in the family may especially upset children. A child may say, as many do at moments of extreme anger, "I wish you were dead." He may wonder, if the person with whom he was angry died later, whether he caused the death. Children don't have a well-developed sense of time. His outburst may have been months before the death, but it may still trouble him.

The patient with ESRD usually has an extended period of time to come to terms with death. He has a chance to settle his estate, get things in order, and prepare himself and his family. I vacillate between gloom and optimism. I've tried to prepare for the worst and enjoy what I can. So far, it's worked for me.

22 The Future

Wouldn't it be nice not to have to dialyze ever again? Wouldn't it be nice to have an implantable, miniature kidney and not to have to wait for a human kidney that matches and not to have to worry whether you'll reject a transplantation? Wouldn't it be nice if kidney disease could be treated so that you'd never get to the point of failure? It's likely that these things will happen in the future. There are some advances that are currently in limited use and that may represent improvements in the way dialysis is done.

One of the problems with hemodialysis is that the artificial kidneys currently in use don't remove all the impurities that are in the blood. Two methods of removing additional impurities are being tested. One is called hemofiltration. It's a modification of standard hemodialysis. When your blood flows into the machine, it's diluted with a special solution and put under very high pressure. This method seems to be particularly useful in controlling high blood pressure.

The other method is called hemoperfusion. It is used in combination with hemodialysis. In this case, your blood passes over a substance, such as charcoal, that draws out additional impurities.

A substitute for hemodialysis and peritoneal dialysis is being tried in the Orient. It may be distasteful to the average American, but it's cheap and simple and, therefore, may be useful in underdeveloped areas. It's called diarrhea therapy. Most of the toxic materials that we need to remove from our bodies enter by mouth and pass to the gut, where they are absorbed and their wastes excreted. The gut, then, is both a membrane and a passageway for wastes. If you can absorb materials through your gut, unwanted substances should be able to be drawn out and passed as waste.

In diarrhea therapy, the patient sits for several hours on a commode and drinks enormous amounts of a special fluid. At first, he produces diarrhea as we know it. Then he produces a clear liquid, which is like a dialysate. It draws out the impurities across the gut wall and washes them out.

Now, there aren't many in the Western world who'd go for this method. But remember, in underdeveloped areas, the choice is diarrhea or death. Remember, too, that this method suggests that ways of using the gut may be developed in the future.

A less unusual form of treatment, which may some day substitute for or supplement dialysis, is the use of sorbents. These are materials taken by mouth that "sponge up" substances you don't want in your blood stream. There has been some foreign research with chemically activated charcoal used in this way. Right now, it seems likely that sorbents will be a supplementary treatment. You'd still need dialysis, but less frequently and for shorter periods of time.

Foods absorbed by the gut are broken down into very small components. For example, proteins are split into amino acids. Some of these products are what become the impurities in your blood. Now suppose someone in a corner of some lab comes up with a substance that would recycle these products, making them useful once again. We wouldn't have impurities to clean out. It's just a thought now, but, what the heck, so was the idea of a flying machine.

A Finnish scientist one day saw cows graze, and he asked himself, "How do cows turn that stuff into more cow, baby cows, and milk?" That is, into protein. Nitrogen, the only source of protein in the cow's diet, is what uremic patients have to remove from the bloodstream. What happens to all that nitrogen? He discovered that the secret was in the soil bacteria that the cows swallowed with their food as they grazed. It turns out that the bacteria have an enzyme that makes nitrogenous substances harmless. Right now, he's working on treating patients with this enzyme with some success. One day you may be taking these enzymes (or eating grass), so don't laugh.

Peritoneal dialysis may become much more popular in the future. Right now, there are experiments with continuous peritoneal dialysis. In this system, dialysate is introduced into the peritoneal cavity (see Chapter 8) and left there for about four hours. Then the patient drains it into a bag and fills up with more dialysate. Each change—five times a day—takes 10 minutes or so. The fifth time, the solution is kept in for eight hours to allow time for sleep. No more hemodialysis or machines. A variation on this method involves implanting a membrane—called a mouse—in the abdomen for constant dialysis. Removal of wastes is slow, but even. There are no drastic fluctuations in body chemistry as with on-and-off conventional dialysis. And, best of all, there's no need to restrict fluids or diet. Sounds intriguing, but I wonder if it swishes when you walk!

At any rate, things keep changing for the better. Survival rates keep improving, and the future looks like fun.